PET FOOD POLITICS

MARION NESTLE

....

PET FOOD POLITICS

The Chihuahua in the Coal Mine

University of California Press

Berkeley   Los Angeles   London

University of California Press, one of the most distinguished university presses
in the United States, enriches lives around the world by advancing scholarship
in the humanities, social sciences, and natural sciences. Its activities are supported
by the UC Press Foundation and by philanthropic contributions from individuals
and institutions. For more information, visit www.ucpress.edu.

University of California Press
Berkeley and Los Angeles, California

University of California Press, Ltd.
London, England

The cartoon on p. 167 appeared in the New Orleans *Times-Picayune,* March 23, 2007.
Steve Kelley Editorial Cartoon © 2007 Steve Kelley. All rights reserved. Used with
permission of Steve Kelley and Creators Syndicate.

Library of Congress Cataloging-in-Publication Data

Nestle, Marion.
    Pet food politics : the Chihuahua in the coal mine / Marion Nestle.
        p.   cm.
    Includes bibliographical references and index.
    ISBN 978-0-520-25781-8 (cloth : alk. paper)
    1. Pets—Feeding and feeds—Contamination—United States.   2. Product
recall—United States.   I. Title.
SF414.N47   2008
363.19'29—dc22   2008003995

Manufactured in the United States of America

17   16   15   14   13   12   11   10   09   08
10   9   8   7   6   5   4   3   2   1

The paper used in this publication meets the minimum requirements of
ANSI/NISO Z39.48–1992 (R 1997) (*Permanence of Paper*).

To Malden Nesheim

CONTENTS

INTRODUCTION

On March 15, 2007, Menu Foods, a pet food manufacturer based in Canada, informed the U.S. Food and Drug Administration (FDA) that the company had decided to issue a massive recall of its products. Something in its foods—later identified as wheat flour laced with melamine—was causing so much damage to the kidneys of cats and dogs that the animals had to be euthanized. The company's decision, announced the next day, led to what was then the largest recall of consumer products ever recorded in the United States.

I had a special interest in this particular food recall. Just one month earlier, I had obtained a contract to co-write a book about pet foods and pet feeding with Dr. Malden Nesheim, the now retired chair of the Department of Nutritional Sciences and provost at Cornell University. Both of us have had long academic careers in human nutrition and our colleagues were surprised by our interest in writing about something as seemingly inconsequential (in their view, not ours) as pet foods. The Menu Foods recall established our project as brilliantly insightful. Even our most skeptical colleagues could see that pet foods were the proverbial canary—in this instance, the Chihuahua—in the coal mine. Contaminated pet foods were early warnings of the safety hazards of globalization.

The pet food recall may have begun with the personal—the tragic loss of beloved cats and dogs—but it quickly transformed into the political. The events that followed in the wake of the recall exposed catastrophic weaknesses in global safety systems not only of food production and distribution but also of consumer products as diverse as toothpaste, tires, and children's toys. Contaminated pet foods revealed the need for immediate efforts—by governments and industries—to correct some of the less desirable consequences of our rapidly globalizing world economy.

By the time the events of the recall drew to a close, it had become apparent that pet foods are just one part of an inextricably linked system of food production, distribution, and consumption, a system that involves farm animals—pigs, chickens, and fish—as well as people. Because the tainted ingredient had been imported from China by a company located in Canada, was used to make pet foods in factories in the United States, and was shipped to venues in South Africa as well as in the United States and Canada, what started out as "merely" a problem for "a few" cats and dogs ended up as an international crisis. Consumers lost confidence in the safety of American food products as well as in those imported from other countries, and for good reason. The pet food recall exposed glaring gaps in the oversight of food safety not only within the United States and at its borders but also within rapidly developing countries like China that produce foods for export.

Overall, the recall revealed that anyone interested in the health of people, food animals, or pets should care deeply about how pet foods are made, used, and regulated. Pet foods, as Dr. Nesheim and I had already surmised, are well worth the attention of anyone, pet lover or not, who cares about matters as seemingly distinct as food safety, health policy, international trade, and the relationship of corporations to government. The pet food recall demonstrated the tight linkages among all such matters.

This book tells the story of one particular failure in food safety systems, from its disclosure in March 2007 to the events that occurred throughout the year that followed. And what a story it is. Although pet foods were not the only foods to be recalled in recent years—contaminated spinach, hamburger, and peanut butter leap to mind—most humans do not feel strong emotional attachments to such foods. Pets are another matter entirely. Pet owners (or guardians, as many prefer) are fully responsible for what their pets eat and are likely to be distressed, if not infuriated, when the foods they have purchased cause their dogs and cats to suffer. In part because of the deep bonds of affection between humans and their pets, the story of the Menu Foods recall becomes one of high drama, worthy of Shakespeare, full as it is of selfishness, greed, cowardice, indifference, irresponsibility, secrecy, and deception, as well as frustration, anger, and grief.

By the time this story came to an end, the governments of China and the United States were promising much needed—and long awaited—reforms of their food safety systems and much better guarantees of oversight of international trade. If the governments really do deliver on their promises, some good may yet emerge from these events. If so, the owner-guardians of pets inadvertently caught up in this crisis may gain some solace from knowing that the sacrifice of their animals was not in vain.

This is a comforting thought. But from the outset the promised reforms have fallen far short of the measures that experts have long advocated to ensure safe food for people, let alone for dogs and cats. We can only hope that the reforms will do some good. To make sure they do, everyone who cares about food issues must continue to advocate for better safety policies for the human food supply—including regulations, inspections, and enforcement—as well as for better nutrition standards and more informative food labels for pet foods. Advocacy for policies good enough to protect pets also means advocacy for policies that protect people.

As the author of two previous books about the politics of food, I cannot overemphasize the need for advocacy. In *Food Politics: How the Food Industry Influences Nutrition and Health* (published by University of California Press in 2002 and updated in 2007), I wrote about how food companies—businesses that produce, process, market, sell, and serve food and beverages—influence what people eat not only through advertising but also through government policies. *Food Politics* emphasizes points that now may seem self-evident but were far less obvious when the book first appeared. Because everyone eats, food affects livelihoods as well as lives. Food elicits substantial interest not only from the companies that produce it and the governments that regulate those companies, but also from stakeholders in the food system: nutrition and health professionals, the media, the public at large, and, of course, advocates.

Because food choices affect sales, companies—national and international—want to be free to sell their products with as little regulation as possible. And because our food supply is increasingly centralized and global, the lack of adequate regulation is an international as well as a domestic problem, one that very much reflects how governments choose to balance corporate against public interests. Thus, food choices and food safety problems fall squarely in the realm of politics. Because these concerns are political, they touch on matters central to the functioning of democratic institutions. The pet food recall constitutes a classic case study of food politics in action and of the role of stakeholders in democratic societies.

Dogs and cats may seem remote from fundamental questions about the functioning of democratic societies, but in this particular instance they were central. As the story unfolds, we will see how food companies and government agencies tended to view pets as "just pets." Owner-guardians, however, view pets as much-loved companions. These sharply divergent stakeholder positions revealed the political aspects of the events to a greater extent than might otherwise have been evident. *Pet Food Politics* explains how advocates for the health of pets exercised their democratic rights as citizens and brought about changes in policies that could bring lasting benefits in health and safety, and not only for pets. The changes also may improve the lives of farm animals and people in the United States as well as in China and other developing countries that export food.

The story told here also illustrates issues discussed in another of my books, *Safe Food: Bacteria, Biotechnology, and Bioterrorism* (University of California Press, 2003). Despite its formidable title, this book is simply about the politics of food safety. The politics of food safety? Food safety would seem to be the least political of food issues, as everyone wants food to be safe. Unsafe food is not only bad for health, it is bad for business. Recalls are expensive, negative publicity hurts sales, and lawsuits are costly. The loss of public trust also must be factored into the cost accounting.

But food safety is political for many of the same reasons discussed in *Food Politics:* economic self-interest, stakeholder differences, and collision of viewpoints. The pet food recall elicits many of the questions that come up in any food safety crisis. Who bears the risk of food safety problems? Who benefits from ignoring them? Who makes the policy decisions? Who controls the food supply? Who pays the costs? These questions are political, and they demand political responses.

I've already mentioned that the pet food recall illustrates the kinds of problems that can occur as a result of today's global food systems. Here is another one: the United States and other industrialized countries make far more food available than is needed by their populations. Overabundant food increases competition in the food industry and forces companies to do everything they can to reduce costs and keep prices low. Intense competition, together with legal obligations to maximize profit, leads food companies to:

- merge into larger, more concentrated, and more centralized units
- outsource food and ingredient production to companies in developing countries
- demand protections for domestic food production that act as barriers to international trade
- pressure governments to make policies and regulations favorable to their interests
- cut corners on matters of food safety

Pet Food Politics explains why anyone who cares about the safety of the food supply—for people, farm animals, or pets—needs to be vigilant in demanding the highest safety standards from food producers and distributors, as well as the strongest possible oversight of food safety from government regulators.

A Note about Methods

This account of the pet food recall and its subsequent events is based on my review of a wide variety of sources, ranging from official government documents to the decidedly unofficial—but, in this case, essential—accounts of Internet bloggers. It was not easy to acquire this information. Because the recalls involved a large number of pet food and food ingredient manufacturing, retailing, distributing, and importing companies in the United States, Canada, and China, many facts about who sold what to whom were proprietary and undisclosed. And because the FDA did not have the authority to order recalls of the contaminated pet foods, agency officials were restricted from publicly identifying companies involved in the production and distribution of the contaminated products, even when the FDA knew who they were. My attempts to obtain more direct information from pet food companies were often thwarted by stonewalling or constrained by the fact that nearly all of them were involved in ongoing litigation. Although some government officials, university researchers, veterinarians, and pet food company scientists were willing to discuss their knowledge of these events with me, most did so only when I agreed not to name them. Our conversations had to be off the record. Consequently, I was not always able to document undisclosed aspects of these events and had to leave some sources unidentified and some crucial questions unanswered.

This account is mostly based on information that is publicly available and supported by documentation. Its events are so evidently important to public debates about democratic institutions that they occupied the front pages of newspapers for months. Indeed, food editors ranked the pet food recall as the most important food story of 2007, one even more prominent than those about recalls of ground beef and peanut butter, the safety of food imported from China, or marketing fast foods to children. The barking of this particular Chihuahua attracted worldwide attention and produced worldwide repercussions. We owe the dogs and cats involved in this episode a debt of gratitude. Read on.

1

....

A RECALL TO BREAK ALL RECORDS

On or about February 20, 2007, a Canadian manufacturer of pet foods, Menu Foods Income Trust, received a call on the toll-free customer service line listed on the labels of the products it manufactures. A customer was calling to complain that a cat had developed kidney problems soon after eating one of the company's foods. A second call with a similar complaint arrived a week later. As is customary practice for dealing with such complaints, the firm contacted the veterinarians who were treating the cats. The veterinarians suggested that the cats, both of which had been adopted as strays, might have wandered off and gotten into something like antifreeze. A third call on March 5 reported the death of a cat from kidney failure but Menu was unable to contact its veterinarian. Two more reports of similarly sick cats came in on March 6 and 7.

While these calls were trickling in, and apparently by coincidence, the company that Menu Foods hires to test the palatability of its pet foods began conducting its routine quarterly taste trials.

Pet food manufacturers order such trials to find out whether cats and dogs are willing to eat foods with new ingredients, and whether the animals prefer to eat that company's foods or those made by competitors. This testing company ran palatability tests for Menu Foods every three months or so. Because some Americans strongly disapprove of animal experimentation (especially when it involves dogs and cats) and are not shy about making their opinions known, the laboratories that do such work tend to keep a low profile. The identity of this particular testing company has not been publicly disclosed.

The anonymous company's palatability testing began on February 27 and involved 40 to 50 cats and dogs in at least three separate concurrent trials. The first trial offered 20 cats a choice of a product made by Menu Foods or one produced by another company. On the third day of that trial, the testing company reported that three of the 20 cats were sick with kidney disease. In the second trial, also involving 20 cats, three were ill with kidney disease, and one was so sick that it had to be euthanized. As it happened, either it or one of the other sick cats was more than 16 years old.

Later, in explaining to Congress why his company was not alarmed by these initial findings, Menu Foods' president and chief executive officer, Paul Henderson, noted that the cats had participated in tests of foods produced by at least two other manufacturers, and that all were at least ten years old, implying that they were susceptible to kidney disease anyway. His company, Henderson told Congress, had no reason to think that its foods were making cats sick.

Nevertheless, Henderson told Congress, "out of an abundance of caution," the company "stepped up" its investigation. It identified several ingredients common to the foods that the sick cats had been eating, among them the amino acids glycine and taurine (normal components of protein), "digest" (a meat-based flavoring ingredient), caramel color, salt, and wheat gluten. Of these, only wheat gluten seemed suspicious. Menu Foods had recently changed suppliers and was getting this ingredient from a new source.

About wheat gluten: this substance is a mixture of proteins extracted from wheat flour by repeatedly washing away the starch. In the human food supply, it is sometimes called wheat meat, vegetarian meat substitute, or seitan. In pet foods, wheat gluten has three functions: it adds protein, binds other ingredients, and thickens gravy-style foods. Recently, the extraction process had become so expensive that most American companies no longer made wheat gluten. By 2006, about 80% of the wheat gluten purchased by American companies came from companies in Europe, Australia, or Asia. That year, American companies bought 14% of their wheat gluten from China, twice the amount purchased just one year earlier.

In November 2006, Menu Foods switched suppliers and began to buy wheat gluten from ChemNutra, a company based in Las Vegas, from which it had previously obtained other pet food ingredients. Alarmed or not, Menu Foods halted shipments from ChemNutra on March 6, and two days later informed that company that there might be a problem with its wheat gluten.

The next day, March 9, the palatability testing company reported that it had been forced to euthanize four sick cats from the first study and two more from the second study, and that nine more cats from the first study were sick. This meant that seven of the 20 cats in the first study were dead—a death rate of

35%. Menu Foods was sufficiently concerned to initiate a serious investigation. It asked the palatability testing company to check the pet foods for substances that could be harmful if present at excessive levels: minerals, heavy metals, antifreeze, vitamin D, fluorine, mold, and microbes. Menu also sent samples of the foods to the Animal Diagnostic Laboratory at Cornell University for analysis but did not mention the deaths or concerns about kidney disease. The company just told the laboratory at Cornell that cats were refusing to eat the foods and asked it to test for pesticides and insecticides. When the tests revealed nothing unusual, Menu sent Cornell more food samples as well as samples of tissues and urine from the sick cats. But the Cornell laboratory found nothing unusual in these samples either.

On March 13, Procter & Gamble (P&G), the large home-products company that owns two high-end brands of pet food, Iams and Eukanuba, informed Menu Foods that it had received calls from three customers about "renal issues" in cats, one of which had died of kidney failure. The cats had become ill soon after eating specific lots of Iams foods manufactured at the Menu Foods' plant in Emporia, Kansas. P&G's in-house veterinarian contacted Menu, learned that wheat gluten was coming from a new supplier, and by March 14 was alarmed enough to have the company suspend production of Iams foods made at that plant. At 8:30 that night, P&G informed Menu that it would be ordering a recall of foods made at the Emporia plant since December 17, 2006—the earliest date of production of the specific Iams products mentioned in consumer complaints to P&G.

The next afternoon, March 15, Menu notified the FDA that something in its products, most likely the wheat gluten, seemed to be causing kidney failure in cats and that the company intended to issue a recall. Finally, on March 16, nearly one month after the first reports of cat deaths, Menu Foods announced a recall of foods made at its plant in Emporia and, as a precaution, those made at its plant in Pennsauken, New Jersey. It chose December 3, 2006, as the starting date because foods mentioned in the consumer complaints to the Menu Foods call number were first produced during that week. The astonishing upshot was that Menu Foods would be pulling from the market more than 60 million cans and small foil pouches of "cuts-and-gravy" style dog and cat foods.

Although this was the largest pet food recall in history—and, indeed, the largest recall of any consumer product recorded at the time—it amounted to just 1% of the totality of canned, pouched, and kibble-style pet foods available on the market. Despite the tiny percentage, the recall surely came as a sharp shock to investors; Menu Foods estimated that this action might cost the company as much as $40 million (Canadian). As we will see, this guess was a substantial underestimate.

But the most profound shock was to pet owners. The recall affected pet foods marketed under the most trusted brand names, all of them made by a company unknown to consumers. Menu Foods, the recall revealed, was the largest North American manufacturer of private-label "wet" pet foods, those packaged in cans or pouches. Its products were widely distributed and sold by supermarkets, mass merchandisers, and pet supply retailers. Indeed, Menu Foods manufactured canned and pouched foods for nearly all—17 of the top 20—North American pet food retailers under a breathtaking array of brand names. Menu's plant in Emporia alone produced 42 brands of cat food and 53 brands of dog food. These ranged from the cheapest brands, such as the Ol' Roy foods sold at Wal-Mart stores, to P&G's premium Iams and Eukanuba labels (the complete list of recalled brands is given in the Appendix). Yet here these brands were, all lumped together in one recall, all made at exactly the same place, all with virtually identical ingredients, and all made by one manufacturer. And at least one of these ingredients was causing cats to die of kidney failure or to become so sick with kidney disease that the animals had to be euthanized.

2

....

A BRIEF HISTORICAL DIGRESSION

The Menu Foods recall was by no means the first time a pet food company was forced to announce publicly that something was so badly wrong with its products that pets could not eat them without risk of harm. Recalls, it seems, are not all that uncommon. When the need for them occurs, companies are supposed to contact the FDA, the agency responsible for regulating food safety, and work with that agency to issue a recall, make sure the product is no longer for sale, and destroy the recalled stocks. Occasionally, the FDA does its own testing of pet food samples and finds evidence of microbial contamination or other hazards. On such occasions, the FDA encourages the companies to voluntarily recall the products.

Note my choice of words. The FDA has to *ask* companies for a *voluntary* recall. At the time of these events, the FDA did not have the authority to order a company to recall hazardous products. All it could do was to encourage the company to take responsibility, warn the public not to buy the products, and alert retailers of the need to remove the products from shelves. As the FDA explains in its written advisories, "There is no statutory authority for recalls. All recalls are therefore voluntary on the part of the recalling firm." An FDA official explained to me that conversations with companies about the need for a recall could sometimes become rather strained. As a last resort, the FDA can threaten to go public with its concerns, but it rarely needs to. In truly extreme cases, the FDA can go to court and argue for injunctions or file criminal charges, but what would be the point? By the time such tedious legal processes could be completed, the products would have long been sold and eaten.

Nevertheless, from 1995 through 2007, the FDA issued a dozen or more warnings to consumers or notices of voluntary recalls of pet foods. Also during those years, the Centers for Disease Control and Prevention (CDC) warned pet owners to avoid feeding a food recalled from the human supply—in this case, peanut butter—to their dogs or cats. And although the company never issued a formal recall, Wal-Mart in 2007 quietly removed some potentially hazardous products from shelves. This collection of incidents is summarized in Table 1. The table also lists one additional recall relevant to this story—a recall of Mars dog and cat foods in Asia in 2004.

As is evident from the table, a number of the pet food recalls were international. They involved products made in Canada, the United States, China, and Thailand, or ingredients imported from China and Chile. Some pet foods recalled in the United States had already been shipped to any number of foreign countries. The recalls affected a wide range of pet foods—those intended for dogs and cats; packaged in cans, pouches, boxes, or bags; and with the contents wet, dry, or frozen raw. Several of

Table 1. Some recalls of pet food products, 1995–2007

Year	Company and Product	Problem
1995	Nature's Recipe/Southwest Pet Products (U.S.): dry dog and cat food	Fungal toxin
1998	Doane Pet Care (U.S.): Ol' Roy,* multiple products	Aflatoxin
1999	Farm Meats (Canada): dog treats made from pig ears	*Salmonella*
	Euro-Can Pet Products (Canada): dog treats made from pig ears, pigskins, pork lungs, beef and pork bone	*Salmonella*
	Sargeant's Pet Products (U.S.): dog treats made from beef trachea	*Salmonella*
2000	Iams (U.S.): dry dog food	Excess methionine (an amino acid)
	Nestlé Purina PetCare (U.S.): Friskies Fancy Feast canned cat food	Not properly retorted (inadequately cooked)
2003	Champion Pet Food (Canada) and Pet Pantry International (U.S.): dry dog food	Possible presence of by-products from a Canadian cow with BSE (mad cow disease)
	Petcurean Pet Nutrition (Canada)/ Merrick Pet Care (U.S.): Go! Natural dog and cat foods	Liver failure due to immune-induced hemolytic anemia of undetermined cause
2004	Effem Foods, a unit of Mars, Inc. (Thailand): Pedigree dog foods, Whiskas cat foods, and various treats sold in 10 Asian countries	Kidney failure of unknown cause (identified in 2007 as melamine-related)
2005	T.W. Enterprises (U.S.): shrimp, salmon, and other dog and cat treats; later extended to all company products	*Salmonella*
	Diamond Pet Foods (U.S.): dog and cat food exported to 29 countries	Aflatoxin from fungus on corn
2006	Simmons Pet Food (U.S.): wet dog foods marketed as Ol' Roy,* American Fare, and several other brands	Flaking of enamel can lining
	Mars (U.S.): Royal Canin dog food	Excess vitamin D

(continued)

Table 1 *(continued)*

Year	Company and Product	Problem
2007	Wild Kitty Cat Food (U.S.): frozen raw cat food	*Salmonella*
	Menu Foods (Canada), American Nutrition (U.S.), and other companies (Canada and U.S.): more than 100 brands of wet and dry dog and cat foods	Melamine and melamine by-products (cyanuric acid)
	Petrapport (U.S.): pig ear dog treats imported from Chile	*Salmonella*
	ConAgra (U.S.): Peter Pan/Great Value peanut butter in human foods[†]	*Salmonella*
	T.W. Enterprises (U.S.) and Aron Pet Food (Canada): Snackers, Health K9, and Bully Chew dog and cat treats	*Salmonella*
	Castleberry Food Products (U.S.): co-packer of Natural Balance Eatables dog foods	Botulism
	Mars (U.S.): Krasdale Gravy and Red Flannel Large Breed Animal Formula dry dog foods	*Salmonella*
	Mars (U.S.): Ol'Roy* dry dog food	*Salmonella*
	Wal-Mart (U.S.): voluntary withdrawal of Pingyang Pet Products chicken jerky strips and Shanghai Bestro Trading chicken jerky dog treats	Cause undetermined
	Bravo! (U.S.): frozen raw dog and cat food (in tubes)	*Salmonella, Listeria*
	Hartz (U.S.): Vitamin Care for Cats	*Salmonella*

Source: FDA. Pet food news releases at www.fda.gov/cvm/petfoods.htm; enforcement report index at www.fda.gov/opacom/Enforce.html.

   *Various companies manufacture Ol' Roy pet foods for Wal-Mart.

   [†]The CDC issued a warning against feeding peanut butter to dogs and cats.

the incidents involved contamination with *Salmonella* bacteria. Even if a particular strain of *Salmonella* is not toxic enough to make animals or people sick, its mere presence is an indicator of fecal contamination and suggests that the foods were produced under conditions of inadequate sanitation. Among this motley collection of recalls, a few offer especially instructive lessons.

Petcurean, 2003

Petcurean Pet Nutrition is a firm based in British Columbia that makes Go! Natural pet foods and markets them as "wholesome foods for a healthy life." In June 2003, Petcurean recruited Merrick Pet Care to manufacture its products in the United States. In October, after hearing complaints of acute liver failure among pets eating its products, Petcurean issued a recall. Eventually, 48 dogs and 10 cats were affected, and clinical investigations suggested that the animals died from liver disease resulting from the effects of immune-mediated hemolytic anemia, a relatively common condition in dogs that occurs when they make antibodies against their own blood cells. This type of anemia has multiple causes. The FDA tested the foods for a large number of probable causes but found none.

But the FDA did find BHA (butylated hydroxyanisole), an antioxidant preservative often used in food products. Agency investigators observed "overformulations" of BHA four to 13 times higher than is usual in some of the foods. But, they said, BHA is not particularly toxic and "no adverse effects would be expected even at these elevated (4–13X) levels." The FDA's unsatisfactory conclusion: "a definitive cause of the ill effects in the dogs and cats has not been determined" and "may never be known."

The sick pets had eaten foods purchased from a retailer in the San Francisco Bay Area, Pet Food Express. This company accounted for 80% of the sales of Go! Natural products in the United States. After the recall, Pet Food Express paid rebates and veterinary bills for customers who had purchased Petcurean products at its stores. As often happens with recalls, litigation followed. But the lack of a known cause of the pet illnesses created a murky legal situation. So did the "manufacturing deviation"; Go! Natural did not list the decidedly unnatural BHA as an ingredient on its product labels.

Pet owners filed class-action suits against Petcurean and Pet Food Express for negligence; these suits were thrown out of court. Pet Food Express sued Petcurean and Merrick for recovery of the costs of the refunds and veterinary care. The case was settled out of court and "resolved in its entirety" in November 2007, four years after the recall. Moral: it is not easy to prove that a pet food causes illness, and litigation over such matters is often a slow process.

Diamond, 2005

Even when the cause can be found, recalls almost always come too late to do any good. Prior to the Menu Foods recall, the largest previous recall involved products made by Diamond Pet Foods. Late in 2005, some of Diamond's dog foods containing corn ingredients were found to be contaminated with aflatoxin, a toxin produced by a fungus, *Aspergillus flavus,* which proliferates on wet grains. This toxin causes liver failure. Perhaps as many as 100 dogs became sick or died from liver disease before the products containing the fungus-infected corn could be identified and recalled. Investigations by the FDA revealed that the company had no record of testing 12 corn shipments for aflatoxin in 2005. Although the company said it had done nothing illegal, it agreed early in 2008 to a $3.1 million settlement of a class-action suit. The fund compensates owners for loss of their dogs, veterinary expenses, the cost of unreturned contaminated food, and attorneys' fees. Here, the lesson has to do with the substantial cost of legal settlements, even relatively small ones.

Mars Petcare, 2007

Federal agencies worry most about *Salmonella* contamination because these bacteria can make people sick—sometimes very sick. What makes *Salmonella* an especially troublesome pathogen is that the bacteria do not necessarily cause cats or dogs to become ill. But people who handle the foods, or who handle animals infected with *Salmonella*, can become sick, especially if they have weakened or immature immune systems. Children and the elderly are at highest risk, a feature that was clearly demonstrated in an outbreak of a particular type of *Salmonella,* "serotype Schwarzengrund," in 2007. Infections with this *Salmonella* species sickened 66 individuals—and 39% of them were infants.

The serotype Schwarzengrund incident illustrates why it is so difficult to establish a link between contaminated pet foods and human illness. Here is how investigators decided that two brands of Mars Petcare dry dog foods—Red Flannel and Krasdale, made at a plant in Everson, Pennsylvania—were likely to be the source of illnesses in pet owners caused by *Salmonella* Schwarzengrund:

- Investigators from the CDC observed that people sick with *Salmonella* Schwarzengrund ("cases") were more likely than those who were not sick ("controls") to have purchased dry dog foods produced by Mars Petcare at a plant in Everson.

- The Pennsylvania health department found *Salmonella* Schwarzengrund in one single swab sample (presumably from among many) taken at the Everson plant.

- The FDA tested Mars Petcare foods made at that plant and found *Salmonella* Schwarzengrund in one previously unopened bag of Red Flannel and in one unopened bag of Krasdale dry dog food. These were the only positive tests among 150 samples from seven brands of Mars Petcare foods.

- CDC investigators isolated *Salmonella* Schwarzengrund from the feces of dogs that had eaten dry dog food (of unreported brands) in the homes of two of the people who became ill.

These pieces of evidence may appear to illustrate a direct chain of *Salmonella* transmission from the factory to the two brands of food to the dogs and then to their owners (factory → dog foods → dogs → owners), but the CDC concluded that "neither of these brands [Red Flannel or Krasdale] has been linked to human illness." This must mean that the investigators could not find a single case of illness in a pet owner living in a house with dogs that had been fed Red Flannel or Krasdale dry food. Nevertheless, perhaps out of caution or fear of litigation, Mars Petcare chose to issue a voluntary recall of those two brands. It is better policy—for reasons of company reputation as well as pet health—to recall suspicious products right away rather than wait until the cause of the problem has been identified.

Wal-Mart, 2007

The Wal-Mart incident explains why it is so important to investigate the cause of illnesses in pets whenever a food product might be involved. Dogs and cats can die suddenly of causes that have nothing at all to do with what they ate and it is not easy to prove that a death is due to something in the animal's food. In the summer following the Menu Foods recall, while problems with products made in China (as I discuss later) were still very much in the news, Wal-Mart received some complaints from customers whose dogs had become ill after eating chicken jerky treats made in China by Pingyang Pet Products or Shanghai Bestro Trading. Although Wal-Mart did not recall the products, it quietly removed the treats from shelves and embarked on its own testing program. The company ran 17 different kinds of tests on the products. A month later, it announced the results. Laboratory tests had identified slight traces of melamine in the two Chinese products. Melamine, an industrial chemical used to make plastic dinnerware and fertilizer, was the substance implicated in the Menu Foods recall that had occurred a few months earlier. This finding raised questions about why Wal-Mart failed to notify customers who might have purchased the products and still had them at home.

Nevertheless, the melamine finding seemed peculiar. The chicken jerky products were not labeled as containing wheat or any other kind of gluten (the ingredients implicated in the earlier recalls), and the amount of melamine was only about 20 milligrams per kilogram (mg/kg), a level unlikely to be harmful on its own. The FDA did its own testing of the jerky products but did not find melamine or any other biological or chemical contaminant. By September, however, veterinarians were warning pet owners that they were seeing an unusual number of cases of dogs becoming ill with Fanconi Syndrome, a rare kidney disease, after eating the jerky treats. Despite the lack of evidence of anything wrong with the products, other companies making or selling them issued guidelines suggesting restrictions on the number of such snacks that could safely be fed to dogs each day. At the time of this writing, the cause of the reported problems was still undetermined.

One alternative explanation is that the products were just fine and the dogs had become ill from other causes. Without investigating the cause of death, it is difficult to distinguish those alternatives and speculation becomes all too easy. This incident demonstrated an important consequence of the Menu Foods recall: the loss of public confidence in commercial pet foods, especially those made in China; in pet foods containing ingredients imported from China; and, because of consumers' general distrust of the company's cost-cutting practices, in those sold by Wal-Mart. The incident also demonstrated how badly companies want to avoid recalls and how much they prefer to find other ways of dealing with such situations.

Wild Kitty, 2007

The FDA can request recalls, but companies do not have to agree to do them. Indeed, they sometimes (perhaps often) balk. The recall of Wild Kitty Cat Food early in 2007 followed an initial balking. The company first refused but later grudgingly agreed to recall frozen raw products that the FDA had found contaminated with *Salmonella*. Wild Kitty argued:

> Considering the millions of cats eating raw diets every day . . . statistically there is zero chance your cat will get salmonellosis [*Salmonella* infection] . . . The salmonella found in Wild Kitty Cat Food is not a result of poor processing, second grade product or bad sanitation . . . There is no way, short of irradiation of all food products, to excluded [*sic*] salmonella from the US food supply . . . We question the FDA's choice of Wild Kitty Cat Food as part of the bioterrorism initiative on pet food safety.

The idea that the beleaguered FDA might consider pet foods priority targets of bioterrorism comes as news, but never mind. And although the risk of *Salmonella* illness in cats is small, it is certainly greater than zero. But *Salmonella* is not an inevitable component of the food supply. When food is contaminated with *Salmonella*, it means that the food must have come in contact with feces at some point, or with equipment or hands that were in contact with feces. The presence of *Salmonella* indicates a breach in basic food safety procedures. Even if pets do not become ill from eating contaminated foods, giving *Salmonella*-infested foods to dogs or cats does not seem like a smart idea. As was evident in the *Salmonella* Schwarzengrund incident, toxic strains can make vulnerable adults and children sick and it makes sense to try to prevent such illnesses.

But it is not difficult to understand why FDA pressures to recall contaminated products would distress pet food companies. Recalls are terrible for public relations and hugely expensive for the companies. From the standpoint of pet safety and consumer confidence, recalls pose yet another problem; they are invariably incomplete. Recalled products remain on shelves long after official warnings have been issued and can continue to make pets sick if owners unwittingly buy them.

In April, one month after the first Menu Foods announcement, the FDA warned pet owners that recalled products might still be on shelves. But, as I later learned, recalled pet foods lingered in stores throughout the year. In December, a veterinary medical journal printed a letter that Dr. Malden Nesheim and I had written about the melamine investigations discussed in Chapters 9 to 11. In response, I received an e-mail message from Dr. William Maslin, a veterinary pathologist at Mississippi State University (and one of the few correspondents willing to be quoted on the record). He wrote:

> We've seen quite a few fatalities in cats and dogs that have ingested the adulterated food and—considering that the cause has been known for some time—continue to see fatalities. You would think that the adulterated food would be off the store shelves by now, but we had a case about two weeks ago in a cat whose owner is a secretary in our own dean's office . . . although the cases should decrease in frequency and may stop, we are still seeing them. And you can quote me on that. I don't know whether adulterated food is still on store shelves or whether individual owners have old food or snacks sitting in their pantries.

Either is a very real possibility. With these many lessons in mind, let's take a look at some of the early events in the Menu Foods recall.

3

....

THE SEQUENCE OF EVENTS

The central questions in any scandal are "What did they know?"
and "When did they know it?" In this case, because so many
companies were involved, each thoroughly committed to protecting its own corporate interests, such questions are especially difficult to answer. As noted in the Introduction, I constructed this
version of events from information gleaned from many sources,
among them contemporary newspaper accounts, FDA press
releases and news conference transcripts, recordings of congressional hearings, company press statements, and, not least, the
Internet postings of bloggers. Based on what I could document
from public sources, Table 2 at the end of this chapter summarizes my best guess at the order in which key events occurred.

One critical question, for example, is why Menu Foods waited
nearly a month after first learning about the cat illnesses to contact the FDA and issue a recall. As it happened, a congressional
hearing addressed this very question. In his testimony at that
hearing, Paul Henderson, the president and chief executive offi-

cer of Menu Foods, blamed the delay on the FDA, research groups, and testing laboratories for taking so long to identify the toxin, as well as on pet owners for their potentially irrational behavior:

> We acted quickly and took appropriate steps under the circumstances . . . It took the FDA, prestigious research organizations and several commercial laboratories many more days to identify melamine in ChemNutra wheat gluten as the source of the problem . . . Based on what was known at the time, there might well have turned out to be no problem with the food, and announcing a recall could have only resulted in unnecessary panic among pet owners . . . Menu placed the interests of pets and pet owners first, so, like our good customer Iams, we decided that, notwithstanding the lack of scientific evidence, we should notify the FDA and begin a voluntary, precautionary recall.

That may sound reasonable, if self-serving, but in response to probing questions from Congress, Mr. Henderson implied that Menu might have waited even longer to issue a recall—or might not have issued one at all—if the company had not been forced to do so by its best customer, Procter & Gamble, the owner of Iams pet foods. In the following exchange, the questioner is Congressman Bart Stupak (Democrat, Michigan):

> STUPAK: But even before you—I don't mean to be argumentative, here—even before you at Menu Foods and the FDA decided to recall, Iams had already told you they would no longer accept your product and they were going to recall all food manufactured by Menu Foods at the Emporia, Kansas, plant, right? So, really, Iams was the first one to really start the ball rolling here, that something was wrong. And I guess maybe what we're getting at here is there's also a corporate responsibility instead of waiting for the FDA. If Iams, the pet food manufacturer, sees

a problem and they're recalling it, I would have hoped that the corporations would have done it without FDA authority. But even with FDA authority, if we could grant that to them, I think we could have maybe limited the scope of the harm caused throughout our country.

HENDERSON: Well, again, relative to the facts as they actually transpired, the conversation that took place with Iams, they essentially shared some information with us. We got together the next day, and essentially in a rather lengthy meeting, both parties exchanged what they knew, being that individually there wasn't enough information to draw conclusions. But together it looked from a circumstantial evidence perspective as if we had the basis for a recall. They opted to recall, we went along. We announced first.

STUPAK: Iams sees the need for a recall, but almost two weeks before that, in your own taste testing lab out of 20 animals, three died and six were dead. That's almost 50 percent. I would think that would cause Menu Foods to be concerned and talk about a recall or what's going on here quicker than wait until Iams forces the issue, and then the FDA, and on and on.

Congressman Stupak's point is that if the FDA had been authorized to order a recall, it might have made a difference. An earlier recall might have prevented illnesses and deaths among cats and dogs fed contaminated products that were still for sale while Menu Foods was trying to identify the toxic contaminant.

Menu announced the recall on March 16. P&G immediately followed with its own recall of 43 Iams and 25 Eukanuba items made at the Menu Foods plant in Emporia. P&G's press release said nothing about the company's role in identifying problems with the foods or in forcing the recall. But its press statement established the pattern that would become common to most pet food recall press releases. These invariably shifted the blame elsewhere, included some version of the pet food seller's mantra ("the health of your pet is our highest priority"), and pointed out that the recall was just precautionary and that the company's other products were perfectly safe. P&G's press release said:

> This voluntary recall is part of a larger product recall by Menu Foods, Inc., a contract manufacturer that makes a small portion of canned and foil pouch "wet" cat foods for Iams and Eukanuba as well as other non-P&G brands . . . P&G Pet Care is taking this proactive step out of an abundance of caution, because the health and well-being of pets is paramount in the mission of Iams and Eukanuba . . . The company regrets any inconvenience to its consumers and retail customers.

So let's pause for a minute and summarize: here we are, just one month into this incident, and already dealing with at least six corporate, institutional, or government entities—Menu Foods, its anonymous palatability testing company, the Cornell University Animal Diagnostic Laboratory, ChemNutra, P&G, and the FDA—as well as the dozens of as yet unnamed companies that owned, put private labels on, or sold the 95 brands of pet foods that were recalled on March 16 in the United States and Canada (see the Appendix). And this was only the beginning.

To help follow what happened next in this exceptionally convoluted story, Figure 1 illustrates the partial chain of production and distribution of the ostensible wheat gluten ingredient that sickened cats and, as we will soon see, dogs. Complicated as it is, this illustration is incomplete, not least because the names of many of the pet food companies involved and the brokers from whom they bought the tainted protein ingredients remain well-kept trade secrets. But just a glance at the diagram makes it clear

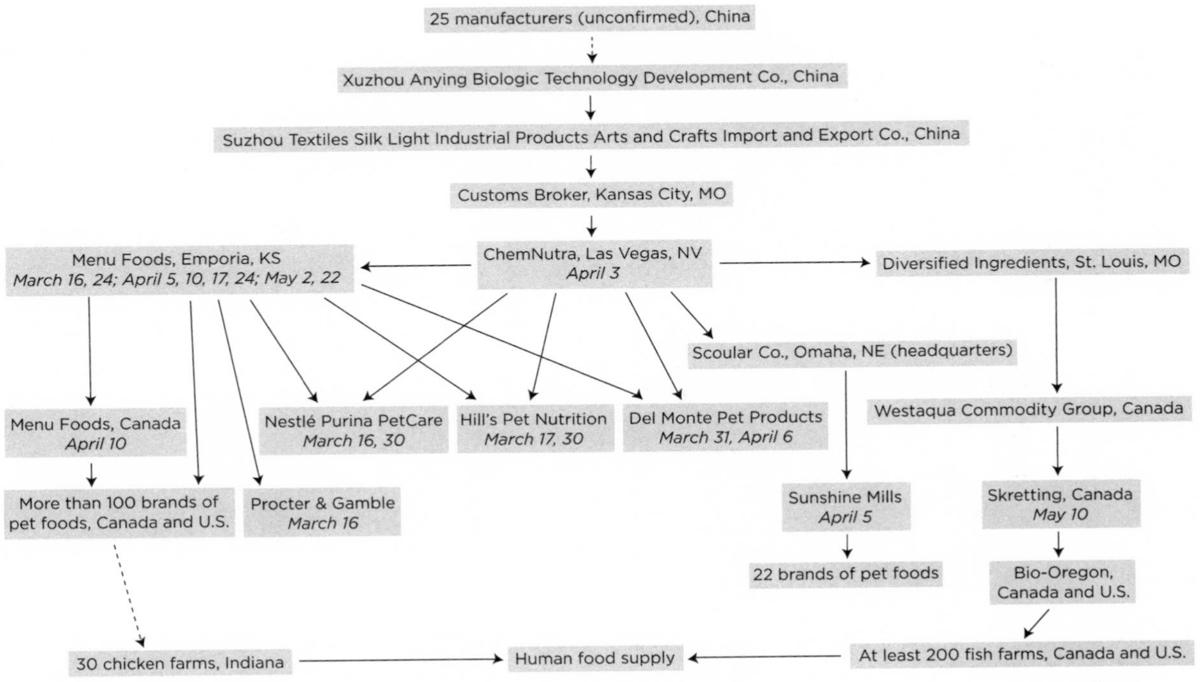

Figure 1. Partial chain of production and distribution of melamine-adulterated wheat flour sold as wheat gluten. Dates in italics refer to the dates of the recall notices listed by the FDA at www.fda.gov/oc/opacom/hottopics/petfood.html. The dotted lines indicate uncertainty about the source of pet food by-products in chicken feed. Companies are located in the United States unless otherwise indicated.

that pet foods are a part—in this instance, a key part—of a large, interconnected, multinational system of food production, distribution, and consumption. In any system this complex, safety problems are easy to overlook and responsibility for them difficult to assign.

Table 2. Timeline of Menu Foods and other melamine-associated
pet food recalls, July 2006–April 2008

Date	Event
2006 (Preliminaries)	
July	Wilbur-Ellis orders rice protein concentrate from Binzhou Futian in China (see Chapter 14).
August	Skretting imports wheat gluten from Chinese company, Xuzhou Anying, to use in fish feed (see Chapter 15).
November	Menu Foods orders wheat gluten from ChemNutra. ChemNutra imports wheat gluten made by Xuzhou Anying.
2007	
January 5	A pet food manufacturer (unnamed) informs ChemNutra that the moisture content of its wheat gluten exceeds specifications.
February, early	Pet food by-products containing Xuzhou Anying wheat gluten are fed to chickens in Indiana.
February 20 or 22	Menu Foods receives complaint about a cat with kidney failure.
February 26	Menu's CFO sells nearly half his units (shares) in the company.
February 27	Palatability testing company (unnamed) begins Menu's routine feeding studies on 40–50 cats and dogs.
February 28	Second customer reports a cat with kidney failure.
March 2	Palatability testing company says three of 20 cats are ill with kidney failure; one is euthanized.
March 5	Third customer reports kidney failure (and death) of a cat. Menu tests foods but finds nothing wrong.
March 6	Fourth customer reports a sick cat. Menu stops shipments of ChemNutra wheat gluten.
March 7	Fifth customer reports a sick cat.
March 8	Menu notifies ChemNutra about possible problem with wheat gluten.

(continued)

Table 2 *(continued)*

Date	Event
March 9	Palatability testing company says seven of 20 cats in its first study are dead and nine are sick; in second study, two of 20 cats are dead. Menu sends food samples to Cornell; says cats refuse the foods.
March 12	Palatability testing company finds nothing wrong with foods.
March 13	Cornell finds nothing wrong with foods. Menu sends tissue and urine samples to Cornell; says foods made cats sick. Iams (P&G) informs Menu that three customers have reported sick cats.
March 14	Tests for antifreeze in wheat gluten are negative. Iams (P&G) tells Menu it will recall cat food made at Menu plant in Emporia, Kansas.
March 15	Owner of five dogs tells Menu one is dead of renal failure and four are sick. Palatability testing company says dogs refuse foods and are ill. Menu notifies FDA it intends to issue recall.
March 16	Menu recalls 60 million units of 42 cat food brands and 53 dog foods made in its Emporia plant between December 3, 2006, and March 6, 2007; estimates cost of recall at $30–$40 million (Canadian). Menu clients issue recalls: P&G Pet Care (March 16), Nestlé Purina PetCare (March 16), Hill's Pet Nutrition (March 17). P&G laboratory receives food samples for testing.
March 17	Menu sets up hotlines to handle consumer queries; callers complain lines are busy.
March 18	Menu hotlines receive 47,000 calls over weekend; callers complain they cannot get through.
March 19	FDA asks ChemNutra for wheat gluten records; holds first press teleconference on recall.
March 20	First lawsuit filed against Menu. FDA reports 14 confirmed pet deaths, nine from testing and five household pets. Pet Connection reports 241 pet deaths.
March 21	More lawsuits filed. New York State scientists identify aminopterin in pet foods.

Table 2 *(continued)*

Date	Event
March 22	P&G scientists identify melamine in food samples. Pet Connection reports 845 deaths.
March 23	P&G scientists inform FDA about melamine finding. Cornell and New York State laboratories announce aminopterin finding. Michigan State University shows photographs of kidney crystals. Menu temporarily closes Emporia plant.
March 24	Menu extends recall to include all cuts-and-gravy varieties. Pet Connection reports 1,541 deaths. Banfield veterinary hospitals report 30% increase in cat kidney failures. P&G scientists discuss melamine finding with Cornell.
March 26	Cornell and Advion BioSciences find melamine—not aminopterin—in wheat gluten and pet foods. Veterinary Information Network reports 104 deaths among 471 sick pets; estimates national pet death toll at 2,000 to 7,000.
March 27	Cornell and Advion BioSciences find melamine in urine and tissues from sick cats. Pet Food Institute recruits public relations firm to manage communications strategy.
March 28	Pet Connection reports 2,237 pet deaths.
March 29	FDA tells ChemNutra its wheat gluten contains melamine.
March 30	FDA says food and tissue samples contain melamine from wheat gluten imported from a Chinese company; does not reveal company name; bans further imports from Xuzhou Anying; orders inspection of all wheat gluten imported from China. Hill's Pet Nutrition and Nestlé Purina PetCare recall products made with wheat gluten obtained from "the same company that also supplied Menu Foods."
March 31	ChemNutra and Xuzhou Anying CEOs meet in China. Pet Connection reports 2,797 deaths (1,546 cats; 1,251 dogs). Del Monte recalls products made with wheat gluten obtained "from a specific manufacturing facility in China" (expands recall on April 6).
April 2	Menu reopens Emporia plant. China denies responsibility for pet deaths. ChemNutra recalls wheat gluten imported from Xuzhou Anying.

(continued)

Table 2 *(continued)*

Date	Event
April 3	American Hog Farm buys salvage from Diamond Pet Foods, co-packer of Natural Balance.
April 4	Wilbur-Ellis receives shipment of rice protein concentrate from Binzhou Futian; finds one sack labeled "melamine."
April 5	FDA names ChemNutra as wheat gluten supplier, says it received 12,000 calls about pet illnesses; gives official number of pet deaths as 16. Menu expands recall to include more brands and a broader range of dates (November 8 to March 6). Sunshine Mills recalls dog biscuits made with wheat gluten "from a specific manufacturing facility in China."
April 6	FDA raises possibility that melamine is a deliberate adulterant.
April 10	Menu Foods expands recall to include products made in its Mississauga, Ontario, plant with wheat gluten shipped to it from Emporia; says reporting delay due to a clerical error.
April 12	Senate holds hearing on pet safety. Pet Food Institute places full-page advertisements in national newspapers; announces formation of an investigative commission. FDA says contaminated pet foods remain on retailers' shelves.
April 13	Natural Balance hears complaints from customers that venison products are making pets sick; suspects melamine in rice protein concentrate. American Hog Farm again buys salvage from Diamond Pet Foods.
April 15	Wilbur-Ellis notifies FDA about April 4 melamine delivery.
April 17	Menu recalls one more dog food brand. Natural Balance confirms melamine in rice protein concentrate; recalls venison products. Royal Canin recalls South African and Namibian pet foods with melamine-contaminated corn gluten.
April 18	FDA confirms melamine in rice protein concentrate; tells California Department of Food and Agriculture that melamine is in the urine of hogs fed salvaged pet foods. Wilbur-Ellis recalls rice protein concentrate.

Table 2 *(continued)*

Date	Event
April 19	FDA says 15,000 calls came in about recall; says Wilbur-Ellis shipped rice protein concentrate to Natural Balance and other unnamed companies (during teleconference, reporter tells FDA that Blue Buffalo is one such company and has just issued recall). Royal Canin issues recall. California officials announce that hogs were fed salvaged pet foods containing melamine/rice protein.
April 20	Scientists from the University of Guelph and Cornell and Michigan State universities identify cyanuric acid in wheat gluten. California quarantines hog farm. Royal Canin recalls pet foods made in Canada. SmartPak issues recall (issues further recalls on April 25 and May 2).
April 23	China gives FDA permission to investigate.
April 24	FDA says it will expand testing of protein ingredients; says use of salvaged pet food to feed farm animals is routine. House of Representatives holds hearing on pet food safety. China seals premises of Binzhou Futian.
April 25	China detains managers of Binzhou Futian and Xuzhou Anying.
April 26	USDA and FDA say meat from 345 hogs fed salvaged pet food with melamine/rice protein are in food supply. American Nutrition recalls 28 products containing rice protein concentrate. Some of its clients—Blue Buffalo and Diamond Pet Foods—issue recalls; accuse American Nutrition of adding rice protein without permission. Chenango Valley Pet Foods recalls foods made with Wilbur-Ellis rice protein. China says it will crack down on food safety violations.
April 27	Sierra Pet Products and Natural Balance recall products made by American Nutrition. Blue Buffalo issues additional recall. Menu says it faces 50 lawsuits. FDA issues import alert; detains all shipments of vegetable proteins from China; searches ChemNutra offices and Menu's Emporia plant; says melamine and related substances were identified in 330 of 750 wheat gluten samples and 27 of 85 rice protein samples, and all positive samples came from Xuzhou Anying and Binzhou Futian.

(continued)

Table 2 *(continued)*

Date	Event
April 28	University of Guelph scientists observe crystal formation when they mix melamine with cyanuric acid. Xuzhou Anying's manager, Mao Lijun, admits melamine was added to wheat flour to make it appear as wheat gluten.
April 30	FDA and USDA say salvaged pet food containing melamine/wheat gluten was fed to chickens in Indiana in February, and 2.7 million broiler chickens entered the human food supply; quarantine 100,000 breeder chickens. *New York Times* reports melamine adulteration in China an open secret.
May 1	FDA says it has received 17,000 consumer complaints about sick pets; of 8,000 calls entered into logging system, half report pet deaths.
May 2	Menu expands recall to include all foods subject to cross-contamination in manufacturing plant; estimates the cost at $40–$45 million (Canadian).
May 3	*New York Times* reports that Xuzhou Anying shipped wheat gluten through Suzhou Textiles to avoid food inspection by Chinese authorities.
May 4	Cereal Byproducts recalls rice protein concentrate sold to three unnamed pet food companies.
May 7	FDA announces results of risk assessment review: risk to humans from melamine is low.
May 8	FDA says both "wheat gluten" and "rice protein concentrate" are actually wheat flour containing melamine and related chemicals. FDA and USDA say pellets with melamine/wheat gluten had been fed to fish in Canada and the United States. China admits Xuzhou Anying and Binzhou Futian sold adulterated ingredients.
May 9	China launches a crackdown on food production facilities.
May 11	Royal Canin recalls dry food lines containing rice protein concentrate.
May 15	FDA and USDA release detained hogs for human consumption.

Table 2 *(continued)*

Date	Event
May 17	Chenango Valley expands recall of foods made with rice protein concentrate.
May 18	USDA releases quarantined poultry for processing; says chickens are safe to eat. Uniscope (Johnstown, CO) notifies the FDA that its feed binding agents contain melamine.
May 21	FDA inspects Uniscope and its supplier, Tembec (Toledo, OH).
May 22	Menu recalls two additional Canadian dog foods that could have been cross-contaminated with wheat gluten.
May 23	Diamond Pet Foods recalls Nutra Nuggets because of possible cross-contamination with rice protein concentrate—the final melamine recall.
May 24	U.S. government asks China to make safer food and to provide data on actions.
May 25	FDA releases report on melamine risk assessment; repeats that risk to human health is low (see May 7).
May 28	Menu says it faces 75 class-action lawsuits.
May 29	Chinese courts sentence Zheng Xiaoyu, former head of state food and drug administration, to death.
May 30	FDA announces that Tembec and Uniscope used melamine to bind feed pellets for livestock, fish, and shrimp.
June 5	China announces overhaul of food safety system.
June 8	FDA alerts international health officials about melamine in fish feed.
June 11	P&G cancels Menu contract to make "cuts-and-gravy" products.
June 29	China vows to reform its food safety system.
July 1	*Los Angeles Times* says owners who don't trust FDA are using private laboratories to test pet foods.
July 10	China executes Zheng Xiaoyu.

(continued)

Table 2 *(continued)*

Date	Event
July 18	President Bush appoints Interagency Working Group on Import Safety.
July 20	China revokes business licenses of Xuzhou Anying and Binzhou Futian.
August 9	Menu sells its South Dakota plant to Mars for $26.3 million; releases Mars from contracts to make Royal Canin and Nutro products.
August 15	P&G cancels all contracts with Menu Foods.
August 17	China issues white paper on food safety; says all food shipments will be tested before export.
August 31	China announces recall system for unsafe food and toys.
September 10	Interagency Working Group on Import Safety issues *Strategic Framework* report.
September 27	President Bush signs Prescription Drug User Fee Act with provisions requiring pet food industry to set ingredient, processing, and labeling standards, monitor pet illnesses, and establish illness notification system.
October 10	Menu estimates cost of recall at $55 million (Canadian); says it faces 100 class-action lawsuits; reduces work force; cuts executive pay.
October 29	China announces nearly 800 arrests of food safety violators; says 80% of foods and 70% of restaurants pass safety inspections.
November 1	China approves draft food safety law.
November 6	White House releases the Interagency Working Group on Import Safety's action plan. FDA issues Food Protection Plan.
December 3	FDA Science Board accepts subcommittee report, *Science and Mission at Risk*.
December 10	China and the U.S. agree to food safety provisions in a new trade agreement.

Table 2 *(continued)*

Date	Event
December 17	Food editors select pet food recalls as the most important food story of the year.
December 20	Menu Foods' unit price is $0.75 (Canadian), down from $7.50 a year earlier.
December 24	China announces new food and drug safety standards.
2008	
January 14	China announces success of its food and drug safety campaign.
February 6	Federal grand jury in Missouri indicts managers and owners of Xuzhou Anying, Suzhou Textiles, and ChemNutra for adulterating wheat gluten and mislabeling it to avoid inspection.
February 13	Menu Foods posts a $62 million (Canadian) loss for 2007.
February 14	FDA identifies Chinese factory as the source of fraudulent heparin associated with 350 cases of human illness and 81 deaths.
February 19	U.S. judicial panel consolidates 120 class-action lawsuits related to the pet food recalls; assigns venue to federal district court in Camden, New Jersey.
April 1	Menu Foods agrees to settle class-action suits.
May 22	Menu Foods settles class-action suits for $24 million.

Sources: Sources are referenced in the notes to relevant chapters. Also see timelines produced by *USA Today,* April 5, 2007, at www.usatoday.com/money/industries/2007-04-05-petfood-timeline-usat_N.htm; *Boston Globe,* April 18, 2007, at www.boston.com/business/specials/pet_food; *Wall Street Journal,* August 19, 2007, at http://online.wsj.com/article_print/SB118606871566686195.html; ChemNutra, April 2007, at www.chemnutra.com/ChemNutra%20Timeline.pdf; Itchmo.com, April 2007, at www.itchmo.com/menu-foods-recall-fact-sheet; and Wikipedia, at http://en.wikipedia.org/wiki/Timeline_of_the_2007_pet_food_recalls.

4

....

WHAT IS MENU FOODS?

I am not surprised that pet owners and the general public had never heard of Menu Foods before the recall. This company does not make any products under its own name. In 2007, Menu Foods was a Canadian company based in Streetsville, Ontario. It was the largest of the North American companies that contracted with pet food companies to make wet pet foods sold under private labels. At the time of the recall, Menu Foods held contracts to make a remarkably large proportion of these products: 75% of the private-label wet pet foods in Canada and more than 40% of all such products sold in the United States.

Another Digression:
The Business of Pet Foods

The pet food industry produced sales of $16.1 billion in 2007, but this amount is minuscule in comparison to the trillion dollars' worth of products and services sold annually by the entire U.S. food and beverage industry. Although a great many companies make pet foods, the industry is dominated by just five; these control about 75% of sales. Nestlé (no relation) is by far the largest player, with a market share of about 32% in 2006 for its Purina PetCare brands. The next largest companies—Mars, Procter & Gamble (Iams), Colgate (Hill's Science Diet), and Del Monte (Milk-Bone and other brands)—hold market shares of 9% to 12% each. For these companies, pet foods are a tiny but profitable sideline. P&G, for example, sold $68 billion worth of household goods in 2006, with only a billion or two coming from pet foods. Even for Nestlé, pet foods brought in just 6% or so of its $78 billion in sales that year.

Commercial pet foods can be dry, as in kibble, or wet. Unless they are meant as treats, both kinds are designed as "complete and balanced," meaning that the foods contain all of the nutrients—calories, proteins, fats, vitamins, and minerals—that a dog or cat needs to stay healthy. Wet pet foods come in cans or pouches. All contain water, but some appear almost solid, while others are "cuts-and-gravy" style, in chunks. Pet foods typically contain mixtures of a long list of ingredients, not necessarily in this order: water or broth; cereals of one kind or another; meat, chicken, or fish by-products and meals; proteins; fats; vitamins and minerals; and a host of food additives that bind the ingredients and add flavor or color. These ingredients must be listed on product labels in order by weight. Here, for example, is the ingredient list for one of the products recalled by Menu Foods, a premium (translation: marketed at a higher price) California Chicken Supreme from Nutro Max Cat Gourmet Classics:

> Chicken broth, chicken, lamb liver, chicken liver, turkey, lamb, food starch, natural flavor, *wheat gluten,* salt, calcium carbonate, carrageenan, sodium polyphosphate, guar gum, potassium chlo-

ride, DL-methionine, taurine, sodium ascorbate (source of vitamin C), beta-carotene, ferrous sulfate, choline chloride, vitamin E supplement, zinc oxide, thiamin mononitrate (vitamin B1), copper proteinate, manganous sulfate, niacin, d-calcium pantothenate, vitamin A supplement, vitamin D3 supplement, pyridoxine hydrochloride, riboflavin supplement, vitamin B12 supplement, folic acid, potassium iodide, biotin, sodium selenite.

Wheat gluten (emphasis added) is the ninth ingredient by weight. In wet pet foods, water or substitutes like chicken broth are usually listed first. Wet foods typically are 74% to 82% water; this particular product is 78% water.

Once past guar gum, the last of the thickeners on the list, the remaining ingredients are essential nutrients—amino acids (the building blocks of protein), vitamins, and minerals. The Association of American Feed Control Officials (AAFCO), an organization of federal and state employees that regulates animal feed, sets nutrient standards for pet foods based on the work of committees of the National Research Council. These committees review research on the nutritional requirements of cats and dogs and suggest appropriate levels of intake, most recently in 2006. Commercial pet foods are formulated to meet AAFCO's minimal standards for nutrient content, although most brands exceed those standards for some if not all required components.

With so many requirements and ingredients, pet foods are not easy to make. They must contain the required amounts of essential nutrients, but putting these nutrients into foods presents a difficult problem: isolated vitamins, minerals, and amino acids do not taste good. Pet food makers must add a range of ingredients to mask the bad taste and make the foods acceptable to pets. Companies, as we have already seen, routinely test pet foods to make sure that animals are willing to eat the products and prefer the tester's foods to those made by competitors.

But makers of pet foods face yet another challenge. Dogs and cats do not buy pet foods. People do. As one dog food maker explained to me, the products have to be nasty enough so a dog will eat them but look and smell good enough for pet owners to want to buy them. Complete and balanced nutrition, acceptable to pets and attractive to owners, is a great deal to demand of one food product. Commercial pet food companies work hard to meet such demands.

The manufacture of wet pet foods presents additional challenges. It requires complicated machinery and lines for mixing, pouring, canning or bagging, cooking, and labeling the products. The equipment and lines are expensive to build and maintain, especially for relatively small production runs. But once a plant is set up to make these products, it can adjust the formulas and production lines to meet any pet food maker's specifications. For most pet food companies, it is easier and less expensive to give up control of production and contract out the making of wet pet foods to "co-packers" such as Menu Foods.

To make the different brands, Menu Foods used 1,300 different recipes, all formulated to AAFCO specifications. Such recipes may differ in proportions of ingredients, but the basic ingredients are much the same. So the recall produced this revelation: the contents of pet foods are much alike, and the most important difference between one brand and another is not nutrition; it is price. This revelation cannot have pleased pet food marketers, who work hard to distinguish their brands and prefer to keep the common source a trade secret. The name and location of Menu Foods did not appear on product labels.

**Table 3. Corporate history of Menu Foods Income Fund,
1971–2008**

Year	Event
1971	Donald B. Green buys pet food plant in Mississauga, Ontario, Canada, from Quaker Oats; establishes Menu Foods.
1977	Robert Bras (formerly with Canadian grocery chain, Loblaws) buys 50% stake in Menu, becomes chairman. Menu buys Pennsauken, New Jersey, factory.
1979	Menu wins contract to produce Loblaws' canned "no-name" pet foods.
1992	Cott Corporation (Canadian soft drink company) buys 44% interest in Menu.
1998	Menu builds plant in Emporia, Kansas.
1999	Cott sells most of its Menu holdings.
2001	Menu buys wet pet food operations of Doane Pet Care.
2002	Robert Bras dies; Serge Darkazanli (formerly with Loblaws) becomes chairman and CEO; company goes public as Menu Foods Income Fund.
2003	Menu buys Procter & Gamble plant in North Sioux City, South Dakota, along with a five-year exclusive supply agreement.

(continued)

Menu Foods' Origins

Menu Foods was founded in 1971 by Donald B. Green, who bought a pet food factory in Mississauga, Ontario, from Quaker Oats. Menu still owned that plant in 2007. The company's history is tightly linked to that of leading Canadian food retailers, as outlined in Table 3. Its next executive, Robert Bras, came to Menu from a position with Loblaws supermarkets, and he negotiated a contract to make private-label canned pet foods for that chain. These "no-name" products proved highly successful, and

Table 3 *(continued)*

Year	Event
2004	Paul Henderson (formerly with Cott) becomes president.
2005	Paul Henderson becomes CEO. Menu reports losses of nearly $55 million (Canadian) and suspends payments to unit holders.
2006	Menu reports revenues of $356 million (Canadian); returns to profitability.
2007	Menu learns of cat deaths (February 20 or 22). CFO sells shares (February 26). Menu issues recall (March 16). P&G cancels cuts-and-gravy orders (June 11), all orders (August 15). Menu unit price falls by 70% (August). Menu reduces work force, cuts executive pay (October 10). Unit price falls by 90% (December).
2008	Menu Foods posts a $62 million (Canadian) loss for 2007; settles class-action suits.

Sources: Gillis C, Kingston A. How one supplier caused a huge crisis, and why it's just the tip of the iceberg. *Macleans,* April 30, 2007, at www.macleans.ca/business/companies/article.jsp?content=20070430_104326_104326. Campbell C. After last spring's pet food scandal, Canada's Menu Foods fights for its life. *Macleans,* September 3, 2007, at www.macleans.ca/business/companies/article.jsp?content=20070903_109055_109055. Other sources are cited in the notes to this and later chapters.

Menu expanded its private-label contract operations during the 1990s. By 2001, after taking over the wet pet food operations of Doane Pet Care, Menu had expanded enough to go public, which it did in 2002. In a method typical of that used by many Canadian corporations at the time, it arranged to be listed on the Toronto Stock Exchange as Menu Foods Income Fund. Organized as an income trust, the company could avoid Canadian taxes by paying profits directly to the owners of its "units," or shares.

In 2003, the restructured company bought a P&G pet food plant in South Dakota and obtained a five-year exclusive contract with that company to manufacture Iams and Eukanuba wet foods. This contract quickly accounted for 11% of Menu Foods' annual income of about $300 million (Canadian) that year. By 2005, however, the company was in trouble. It reported $55 million in losses and had to suspend payments to unit holders. Profitability recovered in 2006 and Menu appeared to be in reasonable financial shape in February 2007, when it learned about the kidney problems in cats eating foods produced by the company.

Menu's Further Financial Difficulties

A few days after hearing about the sick cats—and three weeks before the recall—Menu's chief financial officer sold nearly half his units in the company. In the United States, this action would raise uncomfortable questions about illegal insider trading, but Menu Foods is a trust fund and Canadian at that. Coincidence or not, his action was certainly well timed. The March 16 recall caused a precipitous decline in the company's unit price, as illustrated in Figure 2.

Through much of the previous year, Menu's unit price had held relatively steady at around $7 (Canadian) per unit. After March 16, its value dropped to about $4 per unit. The price fell to $3 after P&G's June 11 cancellation of cuts-and-gravy orders, recovered a bit, but then further declined to $2 when P&G cancelled its entire contract on August 15. A week earlier in August, Mars Petcare extricated itself from its contracts with Menu to manufacture Royal Canin products as well as Nutro brands,

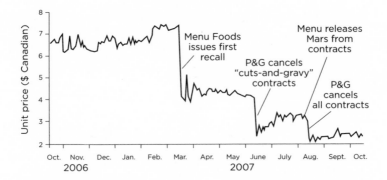

Figure 2. Menu Foods Income Fund unit prices, in Canadian dollars, October 2006 to October 2007. The prices dropped sharply after the first recall on March 16 and again after June 11 and August 15, when Procter & Gamble withdrew its contracts. Mars Petcare also withdrew contracts in August. Source: Stockhouse company snapshots at www.stockhouse.ca/comp_info .asp?view=&Displaycurrency=&symbol=MEW.UN&table=LIST.

which Mars had recently acquired. As part of the extrication plan, Mars bought Menu's plant in South Dakota for $26.3 million (U.S.). But even with that payment, Menu's unit value suffered a 70% loss in the first five months after the recall, and it continued to decline throughout the rest of the year. Beyond these unit price losses, the recall itself ultimately cost about $55 million (Canadian). Still to come were the costs of litigation, which were likely to be considerable. Within just a few months, the company faced dozens of lawsuits. By September, investment analysts were referring to Menu Foods as a "car crash in slow motion."

5

....

MENU'S MUDDLED RESPONSE:
WHAT, WHEN, AND WHERE

Menu Foods gave investors plenty of reasons to lose confidence, starting with its inability to contain the scope of the recall. The company restricted the March 16 recall to products made at its two American plants within certain dates. As Menu gradually uncovered details about the distribution of the wheat gluten, it expanded the number of products that needed to be recalled (the "what"), the dates on which they were produced (the "when"), and the places that produced them (the "where").

The original recall affected cuts-and-gravy products in cans or pouches marketed under 95 labels ("what"), produced between December 3, 2006, and March 6, 2007 ("when"), and manufactured at the company's plants in Emporia, Kansas, and Pennsauken, New Jersey ("where"). Menu expanded the "what" on March 24 to include all cuts-and-gravy products, no matter when or where they were manufactured. On April 5, Menu expanded the "what" again, adding five cat food brands and four dog food brands to the list of recalled products. It also extended the "when," recalling products manufactured as early as November 8, 2006. On April 10, it added 10 more cat foods to the "what" list; this particular recall notice expanded the "where" to products manufactured at its Mississauga plant in Canada. A week later, it added one more "what"—a previously overlooked dog food brand made at the Kansas plant. And on May 2, in the event any cross-contamination had occurred, it recalled all foods made in any plant that had used ChemNutra wheat gluten—44 brands of cat food and 25 brands of dog food. Finally, on May 22, Menu recalled two additional Canadian brands of dog food. By the end of this two-month saga involving eight separate notifications, Menu had recalled 67 brands of cat food and 64 brands of dog food, each of them in multiple varieties, sizes, and packaging formats. According to FDA summaries, the final count involved 18 companies, nearly 200 brands and 5,300 product lines, and more than 60 million individual servings in cans or pouches. The Appendix lists the principal brands recalled, along with an example of recalled product lines within one brand of cat food.

None of this helped pet owners who were left on their own to cope with the lack of information about which brands and products might still be safe to feed their animals. To give just one example: A California pet owner took a cat sick with renal failure to a veterinarian who sent three varieties of Nutro Max food to the University of California veterinary school at Davis for testing. The tests were positive for melamine—the substance that had been identified a week earlier as the probable toxin in the wheat gluten ingredient. Although Nutro had recalled some of its other products, these particular varieties were not on its recall list. Pet owners, understandably, thought Menu Foods—and the pet food companies for which it made products—ought to have known which foods contained wheat gluten and warned everyone not to buy those products. As part of the fallout from the recall, Mars Petcare acquired Nutro Products early in May 2007.

Managing the Crisis

Effective crisis management requires companies to fully disclose everything they know right away, act decisively and compassionately, take their losses, and move on. Guides to managing pet crises in particular—yes, such things exist—instruct companies to put recall plans and teams in place long before they might ever be needed. The guides also tell companies to make it easy for customers to call with complaints, establish human contact as quickly as possible, and deal with complaints promptly and courteously. For reports of sick pets, they advise special handling. Companies should have a veterinarian follow up the cases, send the questionable product for ingredient testing, and, if necessary, send it for palatability testing. One guide advises: "Be prepared to handle the situation in a professional manner and to learn from it; otherwise it will happen again and again."

In the event, Menu failed to rise to the occasion and was widely criticized for its inadequate response. In a poll conducted by *Advertising Age,* 93% of readers judged the company's actions as too little, too late. Menu, they said, violated a fundamental rule of public relations: do not ever, under any circumstances, do anything that might harm children or animals. This rule, said one commentator, "is especially true when you go against one of the most affluent and convergent consumer groups: pet owners."

This commentator was referring to the obvious fact that the owners of dogs and cats adore their animals and are unlikely to remain quiet if something threatens their pets. Pet food companies freely and shamelessly use the attachment of owners to their animals as a marketing tool. Advertisements typically convey the idea that "your dog deserves the best; spare no expense; buy our brand." Menu Foods had been in the pet food business for years and should have known that its customers would be upset—no, outraged—by actions that failed to meet the company's implied or explicit promise to place the health and safety of pets as its highest priority.

In all fairness, it is hard to imagine that any company could have been prepared to deal with a crisis of this magnitude. Menu Foods would have had to hire a battalion of workers just to handle the "make it easy, establish human contact" part of its crisis-management plan. Because it did not sell products to the public under its own name, Menu had never bothered to set up an interactive, consumer-friendly website, and such sites cannot be easily constructed at a moment's notice. Although the company did establish toll-free hotlines, these did not come close to handling the avalanche of questions from customers worried about what to feed their healthy pets or what to do about those that were sick.

The March 16 recall announcement came on a Friday, as such things tend to do. Corporations prefer to announce bad news just before a weekend, when fewer people are paying attention. Nevertheless, Menu's hotlines received 47,000 calls from pet owners over that weekend. By the end of the first week, the company had received more than 200,000 calls.

Menu knew as early as March 9 that something in its foods was likely to be killing cats. By that date, the testing company had reported seven deaths among the 20 cats involved in the first palatability trial. Of the 13 survivors, nine were sick. All told, 16 of the 20 cats eating Menu's products in that trial were affected, a shocking 80%. At the time, Menu Foods had no idea what the problem might be. The testing company had observed odd crystals in the cats' kidneys and urinary tracts, but neither it nor the Cornell laboratory had been able to find anything wrong with the food. Perhaps something else was making the cats sick? For lack of a known cause, Menu continued to dither and did not issue the recall until a week later, and only then under duress.

From the standpoint of pet owners, this "wait and see" approach was nowhere near good enough. As reports of sick cats and dogs multiplied, owners were increasingly frustrated by Menu Foods' uncertainty about which of its products might be harmful, its frequent extensions of the recall, and its apparent disinterest in finding out how many animals might be affected—something pet owners desperately wanted to know.

6

....

THE CAT AND DOG BODY COUNT

The veterinary care system in the United States is not the Centers for Disease Control and Prevention. At the time of the recall, it had no system in place for collecting information from private veterinary practices about illnesses in pets or for disseminating warnings to veterinarians about emerging health hazards. On March 24, the *Sacramento Bee* published an account of the results of Menu's palatability tests, with details of the extent of illnesses and deaths among the cats and dogs involved in those trials. The *Bee* reporter, Carrie Peyton Dahlberg, wrote the account on the basis of an e-mail message sent by the Animal Diagnostic Laboratory at Cornell to veterinary data-sharing lists. One of its recipients, publicly unidentified, forwarded the message to her. Much later, in November, in attempting to verify the details of the testing, my Cornell collaborator, Dr. Malden Nesheim, asked the laboratory for a copy of the original message. Here is the response he received:

Dr. Nesheim—I am reluctant to forward the information that was inappropriately sent to and printed by the Sacramento Bee. That e-mail was intended for professionals in veterinary diagnostics only and should never have been forwarded to the media. I realize that you work in nutrition and are not a reporter, but . . . incidents like that make it very difficult to work with other professionals, especially when you're working for clients who deserve some measure of confidentiality.

This message suggests that the deaths of cats in the palatability tests were a matter of client confidentiality and could not be disclosed even months later, when most of the facts had already been publicly revealed. As seemed all too common throughout these events, protection of business interests took precedence over disclosure of information that might have helped pet owners make informed decisions about what they could feed their animals. That is why the body count—which might seem to be a question of abstract statistical interest—mattered so much to the pet community.

Menu did not publicly disclose the results of the palatability tests until a month after the appearance of the *Sacramento Bee* article, when the company's CEO, Paul Henderson, testified before Congress on April 24. Given the lack of disclosure, the initial reports of cat illnesses and deaths were often inconsistent, as were accounts of whether dogs were affected. On March 19, for example, Menu Foods told the *Wall Street Journal* that nine of 10 deaths it knew about were of cats. For the next several days, newspapers reported the total number of deaths as ranging from 10 to 17, including seven to nine cats involved in the palatability testing. Altogether, 13 to 15 of the dead animals were cats and two to four were dogs. Whatever the actual numbers, the initial deaths seemed higher in cats than in dogs. This made sense. Cats originally were desert animals. They do not need to drink much water and their urine is quite concentrated, a situation that favors the formation of crystals that can block kidney function.

Lacking an official national system for reporting illnesses or deaths, Pet Connection, a web-based group of pet professionals (at www.petconnection.com), stepped into the breach. It asked readers to report illnesses and deaths to its site and also to contact the FDA with that information. Pet Connection's counts rose rapidly: 241 on March 20; 845 on March 22; 1,541 on March 24; 1,841 on March 26; 2,237 on March 28; and 2,447 on March 30. By March 31, Pet Connection had logged 2,797 deaths, 1,546 of cats and 1,251 of dogs.

In providing these counts, Pet Connection pointedly and repeatedly emphasized the uncertainty in its numbers. These, it said at every opportunity, were self-reported, unverified, and unverifiable and could not be distinguished from deaths due to causes other than eating products on the Menu Foods recall list. Pet Connection explained that it was simply attempting to fill the information gap created by the lack of professional, state, and federal systems for monitoring pet health. In collecting this unconfirmed information, Pet Connection demonstrated the need to create a system to address the reporting gap. It also demonstrated the importance of such sites as sources of day-by-day information about the recall that could not be obtained anywhere else at the time.

While all this was happening, veterinarians had to deal with individual cases of sick cats and dogs as best they could. On March 24, Banfield, a large national veterinary practice (owned

in part by Mars Petcare), announced that its member veterinarians had reported a 30% increase in the number of cats they were
seeing with kidney failure, but few deaths. Later, Veterinary Pet
Insurance, a company that provides reimbursement coverage for
veterinary medical bills, calculated that diagnoses of kidney
problems had increased dramatically in March 2007—by 33%
for insured dogs and by 46% for insured cats. This company also
reported that insurance claims for treatment of kidney malfunc-
tion had more than doubled during the period of the recall.
Because neither group collected information systematically, these
figures also are highly uncertain.

On March 26, members of the Veterinary Information Network (VIN), an online forum constituting the "largest group
practice in the world," said its members had reported 104 deaths
among 471 sick animals. VIN surveyed its members and received
1,500 replies, among them reports of 951 sick pets and 313 deaths.
But only about one-third of respondents thought the animals
had eaten recalled foods, and less than 20% were certain the sick
pet had eaten such food. Pressed by Pet Connection to extrapo-
late from these numbers, VIN guessed that the national death
toll should be somewhere in the range of 2,000 to 7,000, and that
veterinary care expenses might cost pet owners $2 million to $20
million. These, of course, were also just guesses. Regardless of
the actual counts—which we now understand will never be
known—the reported illnesses and deaths appeared to be sub-
stantially higher than the official numbers.

By the end of April, both Pet Connection and the FDA had
logged thousands of complaints of illness or death. Table 4 com-
pares their counts. FDA officials were stunned by the number of
complaints. One official told me that FDA hotlines typically

Table 4. Unofficial versus official counts
of pet illnesses and deaths, 2007

Illnesses and deaths	Unofficial: Pet Connection	Official: FDA
Reported illnesses or deaths	14,228	17,000 (8,000 logged)
Reported deaths, cats	2,334	1,950
Reported deaths, dogs	2,249	2,200
Reported deaths, total	4,583	4,150
Confirmed deaths		17 or 18

Sources: Pet Connection, April 30, 2007, at www.petconnection.com/blog/
2007/04; FDA Import Alert #99–29, July 31, 2007.

receive about 20 calls a day with complaints covering the entire
range of consumer products within its regulatory purview.
During the weeks following the recall, the FDA was overwhelmed with hundreds of daily calls about pet foods, more than
the agency had ever gotten about any issue. By the time the calls
stopped, the FDA had received 17,000 or 18,000 calls but had
only been able to enter the details of about 8,000 of them into a
logging system. Of the logged calls, about half reported the
deaths of pets, and these were split fairly evenly among dogs and
cats. The figures reported by Pet Connection were quite similar,
perhaps because pet owners who contacted the site went on to
report the same information to the FDA.

So if the numbers of self-reported deaths were unreliable, what
about those for confirmed deaths? Confirmation requires demonstrating that a pet ate food containing the toxic contaminant and
became ill or died from the effects of eating that contaminant,

neither of which is easy to prove after the fact. Thus, the FDA continued to claim just 17 or 18 confirmed deaths among pets that ate tainted pet food, among them the nine cats that had died during the palatability tests. At a meeting in October, the American Association of Veterinary Laboratory Diagnosticians (AAVLD) reported the results of a survey of "pet food-induced nephrotoxicity [kidney poisoning]" it had conducted from April to June. About 500 veterinarians responded to the survey. In analyzing the responses, the AAVLD identified 347 pets that met its criteria for that diagnosis, among them 235 cats and 112 dogs. Among the animals meeting the criteria, 61% of the cats and 74% of the dogs had died. Death rates were higher among the smaller animals, most likely because they had eaten a greater proportion of contaminated food relative to their body size. The AAVLD investigators admitted that this survey could identify only a "percentage of the cases." How large a percentage? It is not possible to know. These cases also were self-reported, this time by self-selected veterinarians who took the trouble to respond to the survey. Whether their experience was similar to that of non-responding veterinarians is uncertain. Also unknown is the proportion of people who took their sick pets to veterinarians in the first place.

Without a system for following up on such outbreaks, the number of pets caught up in this incident remains uncertain. For a pet owner, one death is too many, and the apparent lack of official interest in determining the toll appeared to be yet another indication of professional, corporate, and government indifference to—or even contempt for—people's deep feelings for the dogs and cats under their care.

7

....

A TOXIC FALSE ALARM: AMINOPTERIN

Menu's reluctance to recall every product that might contain suspicious wheat gluten is understandable for business reasons. Recalls are expensive and generate miserably unfavorable publicity. The company didn't want to issue a recall if it didn't have to. Something—perhaps in the food but perhaps not—was making cats sick, but what could it be? Menu Foods must have suspected right away that something was wrong with the wheat gluten because it ordered shipments to be stopped 10 days before the recall, but attempts by the palatability testing company to identify a toxin had failed.

After hearing about the deaths of nine cats on March 9, Menu sent food, tissue, and urine samples to the Cornell Animal Diagnostic Laboratory for analysis. The Cornell laboratory had been responsible for the rapid identification of aflatoxin as the problem with the foods recalled by Diamond Pet Foods in 2005, and its scientists were equipped to look for such toxins. Although the Cornell laboratory ran hundreds of tests on the samples, it found no evidence of insecticides, pesticides, mold toxins, heavy metals, anti-freeze, or other obvious poisons. At that point, Cornell forwarded the samples to the New York State Food Laboratory, which routinely runs nutrient and toxicology tests on animal feed and has more specialized equipment for doing so. The state laboratory put eight scientists to work looking for harmful chemicals that should not have been present in the foods. After four days of searching, they finally found something: the anti-cancer drug aminopterin.

On Friday, March 23, Cornell and New York State officials held a joint press conference to announce this finding. Aminopterin is an antagonist of folic acid, one of the B vitamins. It is primarily employed as a drug to fight cancer, although it was once thought to be of use as a rat poison. It seemed like a good candidate for the killer of cats because it was known to cause kidney damage in experimental animals. But because it is banned for use as a rat poison in China as well as in the United States, the announcement generated widespread bewilderment.

Pest control experts were skeptical; they had never heard of an incident in which rat poison made its way into the food supply for animals. Could aminopterin poisoning be deliberate? Could this be the work of bioterrorists? FDA officials must have been equally bewildered. They said they had no theory about how aminopterin could have gotten into pet food but could not rule out sabotage.

Cornell spent the weekend trying to duplicate the state laboratory's discovery of aminopterin but failed. The Cornell laboratory and its collaborators could not find traces of aminopterin in the foods. Was aminopterin responsible for the kidney problems in cats? This possibility began to seem increasingly unlikely. But if aminopterin was not responsible for the kidney problems in pets, what was?

8

....

AT LAST THE CULPRIT: MELAMINE

By this time, the FDA had established an emergency operations center to collect information from the 400 people in its 20 district offices and field laboratories who were said to be devoting at least some of their time to gathering samples of pet foods, monitoring how well the recall was working, and collecting consumer complaints. If additional hordes of scientists at pet food companies or universities were trying to find out what had gone wrong, they were not talking about it publicly. Later, P&G scientists said that their laboratory colleagues first heard about problems with Iams pet foods on March 15 and received samples for testing on March 16.

P&G scientists are willing to speak freely, although not on the record, about the work they did to identify melamine because they are justifiably proud of it. Scientists in two P&G research units, central product safety and analytical chemistry, worked as a team to identify the pet food toxin. They began by comparing the chemical composition of foods involved in the recall to that of uncontaminated foods. They spent five days eliminating obvious toxins and attempting to isolate unique chemical impurities in the contaminated foods. Finally, on March 22, they identified a large unique impurity with the spectrophotometer absorption characteristics of melamine. They also identified some melamine by-products, one of them cyanuric acid. Once they were able to isolate and identify the key components, they could see that melamine and cyanuric acid were so plentiful in the wheat gluten that crystals were visible. The crystals looked just like the ones in photographs of kidneys from sick cats that had been posted on the web.

March 22 was a Thursday. The next day, P&G scientists called the FDA and were all set to announce their discovery. But the FDA told them about the aminopterin finding. P&G scientists were quite confident that neither the food nor the wheat gluten contained aminopterin, not least because aminopterin does not form crystals. Nevertheless, Cornell and New York State went ahead with the press conference and announced aminopterin as the toxic contaminant. P&G scientists told me that their colleagues spent the weekend on the telephone trying to convince Cornell that the toxin was melamine, not aminopterin. Cornell sent gluten samples to Advion BioSciences, an analytical laboratory in Ithaca, New York, but Advion found no evidence of aminopterin in any of them.

On Monday, March 26, the FDA sent samples to its Forensic Chemistry Center in Cincinnati with instructions to look for melamine. The next day, the FDA center confirmed the presence of melamine in both the pet foods and the wheat gluten. Once Advion heard about the melamine finding, it too confirmed that the wheat gluten samples contained melamine.

Cornell reported these findings—and its inability to confirm the presence of aminopterin—to the FDA. On March 28, Cornell and Advion identified melamine in urine and tissue samples from the cats that had gotten sick in the palatability testing. Scientists at the University of Guelph in Ontario, Canada, also confirmed these results. The moral: if you know what you are looking for, it is a lot easier to find it. Nobody was expecting to find melamine in pet food, so nobody had been looking for it.

At teleconferences with journalists on March 30 and April 5 to discuss the melamine discovery, FDA officials said they had identified this chemical in the wheat gluten ingredient, in the recalled pet foods, and in kidney and urine samples from the sick cats. Not only was melamine present, but it was present in massive amounts. In answer to a reporter's question, Stephen Sundlof, who was then director of the FDA Center for Veterinary Medicine, explained:

> In the wheat gluten itself we found in some cases [a] very high concentration of melamine. I think the highest one so far has been 6.6% and that's a lot. That means that, you know, getting close to—between 5% and 10% of the product that was sold as wheat gluten was in effect melamine. That's a lot.

Indeed it was. The wheat gluten was so packed with melamine that crystals had formed. But the appearance of the crystals was difficult to explain. They were round and light brown in color and did not look like crystals of pure melamine.

So was the toxin aminopterin, melamine, both, or neither? Scientific reputations were at stake. The commissioner of the New York State Department of Agriculture and Markets defended his agency's work: "We stand confident in our finding of

Aminopterin and know of at least one other laboratory that has confirmed its presence, the University of Guelph's Animal Health Laboratory in Canada" (perhaps, but Guelph reported finding melamine).

Regardless, melamine seemed like a surprising candidate for a pet poison. Nobody at Cornell, New York State, or the FDA could understand how melamine alone could be responsible for the observed symptoms. Their information about melamine toxicity suggested that only very large amounts caused problems in rats and mice. Toxicologists generally considered melamine to be "slightly toxic" to rats and mice, and by analogy, nowhere near toxic enough to kill a larger animal such as a cat. But the effects of melamine had never actually been studied in cats. The FDA mentioned one study of melamine in dogs, but this was an old one, from 1945, that found no harmful effects beyond increased urine output. Although FDA officials did not know how or why melamine might be toxic, they said they were no longer concerned about aminopterin. They would now focus on melamine as the most likely cause of kidney failure in the sick cats.

At this point, the obvious experiment to do would be to feed melamine to cats and dogs and see what, if anything, increasing amounts of the chemical might do to the animals' kidneys. If scientists were doing such experiments—and, as we will see, some were—they were doing them quietly. Experiments on cats and dogs are governed by the Animal Welfare Act of 1966, which requires animals used in research to be treated and housed humanely. Subsequent amendments require researchers to take steps to minimize pain and distress in experimental animals and to consider alternative procedures whenever possible. Scientists conducting animal studies must have their experiments approved in advance by Institutional Animal Care and Use Committees, similar to the Institutional Review Boards that oversee human research. An experiment likely to cause the death of cats or dogs is not something to be approved lightly. Such experiments would be against company policy at P&G, for example. The former dean of a veterinary college told me that his institution would not do a study of melamine in cats because ethical standards precluded experiments certain to cause harm to animals. As another veterinarian explained, "Because of a dearth of past studies on melamine exposure in dogs and cats, the only way to know for sure if it could cause the outbreak would be to feed the compound to those animals . . . That's not an option."

In Chapter 12, I describe the melamine experiments that must have been in progress at that time at the University of California at Davis, but the results of those studies did not appear until November. Without direct information, and on the basis of the earlier research done on rats and mice, officials assumed that melamine was not particularly harmful and were puzzled by its presence in wheat gluten, as well as by its association with the kidney problems in animals eating pet foods on the recall list.

But—and in this case the qualification is a big one—the presence of melamine in wheat gluten should not have come as a surprise to anyone, and neither should the harmful effects of melamine on the kidneys of cats and dogs. To recognize the use and effects of melamine, however, veterinarians and the FDA would have needed to know about studies done decades earlier, well beyond the reach of quick Internet searches. Although their work had apparently been overlooked or forgotten, researchers in the 1960s and 1970s had systematically studied the deliberate use of melamine as an additive to animal feed, as well as the fraudulent use of melamine as an adulterant. These old studies demonstrated that doses of melamine similar to those likely to have been present in the recalled pet foods caused crystals to form and damaged the kidneys of sheep and cattle. They are worth revisiting. Let's begin with experiments designed to demonstrate the value of melamine as a legitimate feed additive.

9

....

MELAMINE:
A SOURCE OF DIETARY NITROGEN

Any old-timer familiar with the history of farm feeds in the United States could guess right away why melamine was added to wheat gluten and why its addition was likely to be anything but accidental. Melamine is an industrial chemical which, when mixed with formaldehyde, forms polymers that can be made into hard plastic dinnerware. This process generates wastewater containing melamine and its by-products, one of which is a related chemical, cyanuric acid. To clean the wastewater and allow it to be recycled, these compounds are reconstituted into "scrap" containing a mix of melamine, cyanuric acid, and other melamine by-products. Because the constituent chemicals contain nitrogen, melamine scrap can be used for fertilizer or for other nitrogen-requiring purposes, legal or not.

The nitrogen in melamine and melamine scrap makes these chemicals excellent candidates for additives—legitimate and fraudulent—to animal feed. As shown in Figure 3, melamine (on the left) is a small molecule that contains six nitrogen atoms. These

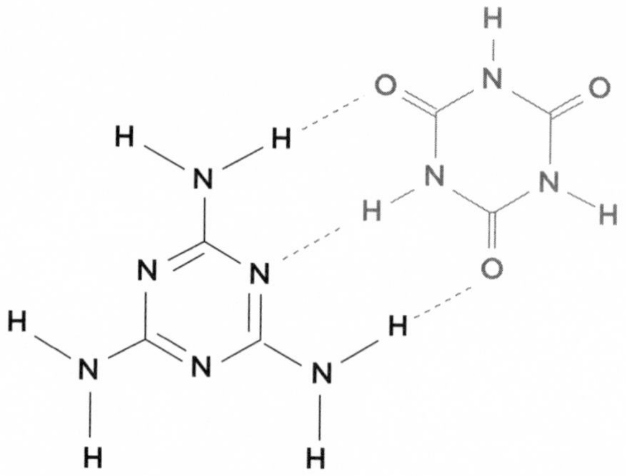

Figure 3. Chemical structures of melamine (left) and cyanuric acid (right). N is nitrogen, H is hydrogen, O is oxygen. Carbons are not shown but are at points where three lines come together. Melamine contains six nitrogen atoms; cyanuric acid contains three. The dotted lines show how melamine and cyanuric acid can link through hydrogen bonds. Such complexes can further link into large crystal structures. The structure shown here comes from Wikipedia, at http://en.wikipedia.org/wiki/Melamine. For crystal-forming complexes, see Xu W, et al. Cyanuric acid and melamine on Au(111): structure and energetics of hydrogen-bonded networks. *Small* 2007;3:854–858.

give melamine a nitrogen content that is 66.6% by weight, making it an unusually good source of an element that is otherwise scarce and expensive. Cyanuric acid (on the right in Figure 3) is 32% nitrogen. That's half the percentage in melamine but considerably higher than the 16% in protein. In case you are wondering, the remaining atoms are carbon, hydrogen, and oxygen.

Melamine and cyanuric acid are "non-protein" sources of nitrogen; they are not amino acids, the building blocks of protein. But when added to animal feed, the chemicals make the feed appear to contain large amounts of protein whether it does or not. This is because feed officials still measure the protein in animal feed using the old-fashioned but reliable and inexpensive Kjeldahl method, which tests for the amount of nitrogen present. It used to be hard to measure the amount of protein in food directly, so scientists just measured nitrogen and multiplied that amount by a correction factor that accounts for the percentage of nitrogen in protein. For most proteins, the correction factor is nitrogen times 6.25. For wheat protein—wheat gluten—the factor is 5.7, because wheat proteins contain less nitrogen than other protein sources. The point of all this is that adding a non-protein source of nitrogen like melamine or cyanuric acid to a farm feed boosts its apparent—but not real—protein content.

Melamine is cheap, but wheat gluten is expensive, not least because its protein content is 75%. Because the official feed assay method can't tell the difference between one source of nitrogen and another, unscrupulous producers can add melamine to wheat flour and make the concoction appear as if it contains 75% protein. They can sell wheat flour as expensive wheat gluten (or, as discussed later, rice protein concentrate). And they can get away with it as long as nobody checks, which in this instance nobody did. Believing that it was buying wheat gluten, Menu Foods bought melamine-adulterated wheat flour from Chem-Nutra, which ChemNutra—also believing it was buying wheat gluten—imported from China. The false wheat gluten most likely contained only the amount of protein typically present in wheat flour—about 10%.

Wheat gluten may seem ripe for fraud, but the honest addition of nitrogen-containing chemicals to animal feed (sometimes with equally bad results) has a long history. In the 1920s, for example, bakers began to use a nitrogen-containing chemical, agene, to speed up the bleaching of white flour. But when dogs ate biscuits made from agene-treated flour, they came down with a condition called canine hysteria, fright fits, or running fits. Agene worked fine as a bleaching agent but by the 1940s was known to be so toxic that its use had to be discontinued.

As noted by the FDA, scientists in 1945 tried to find out whether melamine could be used as a diuretic to increase urinary output in dogs. They fed dogs a dose of melamine equivalent to about 120 milligrams per kilogram (mg/kg) of body weight. A kilogram is 2.2 pounds, so this dose was about 55 mg/pound. As I will explain, a dose of 120 mg/kg is well below the level of melamine that, acting by itself, is likely to cause kidney problems in cats or dogs. Even so, the investigators in 1945 observed that the dogs excreted melamine crystals in their urine. Besides the occasional crystals and the greater volume of urine, the dogs showed no adverse signs.

Deliberate Feed Additives:
Non-Protein Nitrogen

Adding cheap, non-protein nitrogen to the feed of ruminant animals makes sense under some circumstances. Cattle, sheep, and other such animals house billions of bacteria in their rumens, the compartment of their stomachs where bacterial fermentation occurs. As long as the animals are fed a good source of carbohydrate—high-quality hay, for example—the rumen bacteria are quite capable of combining carbohydrate sugars and non-protein nitrogen to make normal amino acids. Cows and sheep can use these amino acids to construct their own body proteins. Decades ago, animal scientists wondered whether melamine and its by-products, cyanuric acid among them, could be useful—and wonderfully inexpensive—sources of non-protein nitrogen to feed ruminants.

Beginning in the early 1960s, investigators in South Africa studied the ability of sheep to use cyanuric acid as a source of nitrogen. Cyanuric acid worked well for this purpose and caused no harm to the sheep, even at doses as stunningly high as 3,300 mg/kg. One of these scientists, H. I. Mackenzie, wondered if melamine—with twice the nitrogen content of cyanuric acid—would work even better. He gave sheep single doses of melamine ranging from 10 to 40 grams without noticeable ill effects. But when he fed doses of 10 or 20 grams of melamine per day for a month or more, the sheep that were fed low-quality hay refused their food, lost weight, and became very sick. Some of them died. The doses that caused these problems were high; they ranged from 275 to 550 mg/kg. Mackenzie did not autopsy the dead sheep. But his report refers to a previous study done by a South African master's student as a thesis project. Apparently, that student used much higher doses of melamine—50 to 70 grams per day per sheep. At such high levels, melamine killed the sheep within six days as a result of substantial damage to various organs, particularly the kidneys.

Clark's Sheep Studies

At this point, investigators knew about the effects of melamine at several dose levels. The 1945 dog study said a dose of 120 mg/kg caused crystal formation but no other harm. Mackenzie reported that chronic doses above 275 mg/kg caused sheep fed low-quality hay to refuse their feed or die. The master's thesis said that doses of 1,000 mg/kg or more would kill sheep outright, but Mackenzie's work indicated that sheep could survive a single dose this high. So what was a safe dose to feed sheep?

Another South African scientist, R. Clark, tried to resolve this question. He decided to repeat Mackenzie's single-dose studies in a slightly different way. His experiment was to give a large single dose of melamine to one sheep at a time, starting with 100 grams, see what happened, and then try again with a lower dose until he could find a level of intake that would do no harm. In these experiments, he administered the high doses through a fistula, a permanent opening from the outside into the animal's stomach. On the basis of Mackenzie's studies, he must have guessed that the highest doses would kill the sheep. Today, a study like this one might encounter some trouble getting through animal care committees, especially because Clark's experiments began with the highest rather than the lowest dose. But he was running these studies in 1966, long before animal experiments were subject to much in the way of regulation.

Table 5 presents Clark's results. A single dose of 100, 50, or 25 grams of melamine killed each of the sheep on which it was tested within one to three weeks. At a dose of just 10 grams per day (263 mg/kg), two of three sheep died within a month but the third survived without showing any adverse effects. When lower doses were fed to sheep, the animals refused their food—a sure sign of illness—especially when water was restricted, but they survived.

Clark's studies suggested that doses of melamine above 250 mg/kg (115 mg/pound) could kill some—but not all—sheep in a few weeks. The deaths, Clark said, resulted from melamine crystals that were blocking the kidney tubules. While the sheep

Table 5. Results of Clark's melamine toxicology studies in sheep, 1966

No. of Animals in the Experiment	Melamine Dose	Result	Melamine Dose/Kg Body Weight*
1 sheep	100 g, single dose, by fistula	Died within 10 days[†]	2,175 mg/kg
1 sheep	50 g/day, by fistula	Died on day 7[†]	1,350 mg/kg
1 sheep	25 g/day, by fistula	Refused food day 15; died on day 18[†]	510 mg/kg
3 sheep	10 g/day, by fistula	1 died on day 16;[†] 1 died on day 31;[†] 1 unaffected	263 mg/kg
3 sheep	7 g fed in 50 g cornmeal, water restricted to 600 ml/day, 6 weeks	Refused food; no other adverse effects	16–165 mg/kg
2 groups of 3 sheep	7 g fed in 50 g cornmeal, 6 weeks; one group water-restricted every other day	No adverse effects	140–165 mg/kg

Source: Clark R. Melamine crystals in sheep. *Journal of the South African Veterinary Medical Association* 1966;37:349–351.

*The weights of some of the sheep are given in the paper; these average 38 kg. Weights not given are estimated to be 38 kg.

[†]Due to kidney crystals and kidney damage.

were still alive, Clark could see white crystals of melamine forming in their excreted urine as soon as it cooled. The crystals were so profuse that he could see "aggregates of crystals . . . hanging from the prepuce of sheep which were receiving higher doses of melamine."

At lower doses, the effects of melamine appeared to be all or none. Some sheep became sick when fed melamine in amounts at or below 250 mg/kg, but other sheep did just fine. Clark's understated conclusion: "In view of the danger of crystalluria [crystals in the urine], melamine would *not* appear to be a promising supplement to rations for sheep" (my emphasis).

Twelve years later, American scientists, aware of the successful use of cyanuric acid as a nitrogen supplement in sheep but apparently unaware of the toxicity studies (their paper does not cite references to the melamine studies of Mackenzie or Clark), fed melamine to six cattle. Although the dose was low—about 100 mg/kg (45 mg/pound)—four of the cattle consistently refused to eat the feed and all excreted most of the nitrogen in their urine. Melamine, they concluded, was not a good source of nitrogen for cattle. The investigators speculated that melamine might be breaking down into some kind of metabolic by-product responsible for the kidney damage in cattle that had been reported previously by other researchers.

By the late 1970s, higher doses of melamine were known to cause kidney damage, especially if food and water were restricted, and even low doses could put sheep and cattle off their feed. The susceptibility of ruminants like sheep or cattle to the effects of melamine might depend on the kinds of bacteria inhabiting their rumens. Several bacterial species are capable of converting melamine to by-products such as cyanuric acid. Rumens are loaded with bacteria and it is quite possible that some could metabolize melamine. And as we will soon see, mixtures of melamine and cyanuric acid at very low doses can form crystals capable of blocking kidney function.

10

....

MELAMINE: A FRAUDULENT ADULTERANT, BUT PUZZLING

Decades ago, whatever might have been known about the dangers of melamine as a source of non-protein nitrogen did not stop anyone from using it as an adulterant. Indeed, its use for fraudulent purposes was so common in the 1970s that Italian investigators were inspired to develop assay methods to test for the mellifluous "melammina" in meat by-product meals intended as animal feed. Once the scientists had worked out the methods, they used the new tests to examine fish meal products. They quickly identified melamine in more than half—56%—of the fish meal samples they examined. The Italian scientists concluded that melamine adulteration was so widespread that anyone who planned to use meat meal or fish meal as an ingredient in animal feed should assume that the meals contained melamine. Their recommendation: all feed ingredients should be examined for melamine—using their tests, of course—to discourage this fraudulent practice.

To summarize, by the early 1980s, published reports indicated that melamine was a frequent adulterant of fish meal, and that doses as low as 100 mg/kg (45 mg/pound) could cause animals to refuse food and lose weight. At somewhat higher doses, animals formed melamine crystals in their kidneys and urinary tracts, particularly if their diets were deficient and they were not drinking much water. At doses up to 250 mg/kg (115 mg/pound), melamine could be lethal to some, although not all, animals. And at doses above 250 mg/kg, melamine crystals were so abundant that they blocked kidney tubules and killed sheep.

But these reports were published in foreign or otherwise obscure agricultural journals, and citations to such old studies do not immediately pop up in modern Internet searches. An abstract of Clark's sheep study was available online, but it did not explain why Clark had done the study in the first place. To answer this question, I had to find the complete paper and the others related to early melamine adulteration in the tedious, old-fashioned, pre-electronic way. This involved time-consuming visits to libraries, searches through old bound journals, requests and patient waits for interlibrary loans, and repeats of this process while sequentially tracing reference lists back to their earliest original sources.

Given the extensive research and time required to find these papers, it is not so surprising that experts caught up in the recall seemed baffled by the association of melamine in pet food with kidney failure in cats. The crystals in the cats' kidneys did not look like melamine crystals and the available literature suggested that melamine was not especially toxic to rats and mice even at very high doses. In the May 1 FDA teleconference with journalists, for example, Dr. David Acheson, who had just that day been appointed to a new position as the FDA's assistant commissioner for food protection, said:

There's a real absence of toxicity data on melamine other than some somewhat old studies in rats. They do indicate that very, very high levels of all ingestion of melamine can lead to significant illness in the rats in the form of bladder stones and ultimately cancer. That's way higher than any of the levels that we've seen ingested by the animals. So it begs the question then what was going on . . . it's probably some sort of combination effect of melamine plus some of the melamine-related compound [cyanuric acid] that is actually what's causing the toxicity.

It is not that the FDA was ignorant of the sheep studies. FDA officials just didn't find them relevant. In June, in response to a query from the *New Scientist,* which had just published a letter about the Clark study, the FDA said: "We are aware of that study and the melamine used was at an extremely high level. We have never said that melamine was harmless to pets."

More surprising is that the sheep and cattle studies also seemed irrelevant to the researchers who conducted a federally sponsored review of the toxicity of melamine, published in May. That review had been commissioned by the FDA to reassure the public that meat from pigs, chickens, and fish that had been fed melamine-tainted proteins or pet food would be safe for people to eat (see Chapter 15). The report firmly states that "the toxicity of melamine to mammals is low" and suggests that crystallization only takes place at high dose levels. The report gives few citations (just six) and these are mostly reviews that refer to some of the studies done on dogs but largely discuss those done on rats and mice. Based on the rodent studies, the review concluded that doses of melamine below 63 mg/kg (30 mg/pound) were most definitely safe. The review said higher doses also could be safe but did not mention what the highest safe dose might be.

We will never know whether earlier suspicion of melamine would have hastened the recall or improved veterinary care of the sick dogs and cats, but the lessons are clear. The old experiments on animal feeding are worth reading, it's best to read entire papers and not just their abstracts, and libraries still have much to offer that the Internet cannot. But even if the toxicology review had discussed the earlier studies, it still might not have mentioned how much melamine—and cyanuric acid—dogs and cats were consuming from the tainted pet foods. The amounts of melamine and cyanuric acid in the pet foods appeared to be another one of those closely guarded secrets, as addressed in the next chapter.

11

....

HOW MUCH MELAMINE
WAS IN THE PET FOOD?

If 63 mg/kg is definitely safe and, as we have seen, 250 mg/kg is not safe for some proportion of animals, just how much melamine were cats and dogs consuming when they ate the adulterated pet foods? If the FDA or pet food companies were measuring the amounts of melamine in the various brands of pet foods, they were not disclosing what they seemed to be treating as another trade secret. But FDA officials did give some clues. As I mentioned earlier, during the FDA teleconference on April 5, Dr. Stephen Sundlof told reporters that melamine was present in the wheat gluten at a concentration of 5% to 10%. In answer to questions during the teleconference of May 3, Dr. David Acheson extended the range downward. He said the amount of melamine in the Chinese wheat gluten ranged from 0.2% to 9%. He provided one other clue: the amount of wheat gluten in the pet food ranged from 5% to 10%. During the May 30 FDA teleconference, however, Acheson extended the melamine range upward;

this time, he said the Chinese wheat gluten contained up to 20% melamine. To summarize the FDA's various statements:

- Wheat gluten in pet food ranged from 5% to 10%.
- Melamine in wheat gluten ranged widely from 0.2% to 20%.

So let's do some guesswork based on these figures, starting with the worst possible scenario: wheat gluten comprises 10% of the weight of the dry ingredients in pet foods, and melamine comprises 20% of the weight of wheat gluten. In this worst case, 100 grams of dry pet food ingredients could contain as much as 10 grams of wheat gluten, and that amount of wheat gluten could contain as much as 2 grams (2,000 mg) of melamine. A hundred grams (a little over 3 ounces) of dry pet food ingredients is about what a large cat or a small dog, one weighing 5 kg (11 pounds), might consume in a day. Dividing 2,000 mg by 5 kg gives a dose of melamine of 400 mg/kg. This amount is well above the 250 mg/kg that made some of the sheep sick and is more than six times the 63 mg/kg "safe" dose given in the FDA's toxicology report. If the pets were old, sick, or not drinking much water, even lower doses of melamine—all by itself—might have caused kidney damage.

But, as it happened, melamine was not acting alone. It had company.

12

....

MYSTERY SOLVED: CYANURIC ACID

By April 20, three groups of scientists—from the University of Guelph and from Cornell and Michigan State universities—had identified yet another compound that was not supposed to be in the wheat gluten: cyanuric acid. Cyanuric acid, as noted earlier, is a by-product of melamine. It is used industrially to stabilize solutions for chlorinating swimming pools and hot tubs and can be made either through chemical processes or the action of bacteria. Pure cyanuric acid, according to South African scientists of the 1960s, was not at all toxic when fed to sheep even at enormous doses, and it worked well as a source of nitrogen in the diets of those animals. But now we know through three kinds of scientific studies—laboratory, tissue sample, and animal—that the combination of melamine and cyanuric acid quickly forms crystals. As a result, we can be fairly certain about what happened to cats and dogs unfortunate enough to be fed pet foods contaminated with these chemicals.

Laboratory Experiments

On April 28, scientists at the University of Guelph reported the results of a mixing experiment. When they mixed equal parts of melamine and cyanuric acid together, the chemicals immediately formed round, brownish crystals just like the ones seen in the urinary tracts of the dead cats. This was an impressive finding, but not unexpected. Chemists had shown earlier that melamine and cyanuric acid readily form hydrogen-bonded complexes and networks (see Chapter 9). Such crystals dissolve in acid but might well be expected to crystallize out of solution under the neutral or only slightly acidic conditions found in kidney tubules.

Tissue Sample Analyses

Test tube experiments suggest what might happen in an animal's body but do not constitute proof. To establish what really happened requires examination of samples from the animals themselves. Scientists at the University of Georgia's Veterinary Diagnostic Laboratory were sent tissue samples from the bodies of 14 cats and dogs that had died of this new diagnosis—"pet food–induced kidney failure"—between February and June 2007.

To make their studies even more informative, the Georgia scientists also received samples from the bodies of two dogs that died in 2004 during a mysterious outbreak of kidney failure that occurred in Asia. The Asian outbreak affected about 6,000 dogs and an unstated number of cats. The animals had eaten Mars pet foods—Pedigree dog foods and Whiskas cat foods—manufactured at a particular plant in Thailand and sold throughout at least 10 Southeast Asian countries. Asian scientists had described the unusual kidney symptoms seen in the dogs but had not been able to identify what caused them.

The Georgia investigators found signs of acute kidney failure in all 16 of the animals, all of which had crystals in their kidneys. They tested kidney tissues from six of the animals for melamine and cyanuric acid and found both chemicals in samples from all six. They also found both chemicals in the kidney crystals. In addition to demonstrating that crystals of melamine and cyanuric acid were the likely cause of kidney failure in these animals, the investigators solved the riddle of the Asian kidney disease outbreak. The tissue samples from dogs in the 2004 Asian outbreak looked exactly like tissue samples collected in the 2007 Menu Foods outbreak in the United States, suggesting that the Asian dogs also had died of pet food–induced kidney failure. This observation, of course, meant that the Asian outbreak was most likely caused by the fraudulent addition of melamine and cyanuric acid to some ingredient in the pet foods made in Thailand in 2004.

Animal Experiments

At this point, it might seem as though whatever needed to be known about the toxicity of melamine and cyanuric acid was known well enough. Melamine, perhaps alone at high doses, but certainly in combination with cyanuric acid at any dose, is bad news for cats and dogs unlucky enough to be fed it. Nevertheless, veterinary scientists were troubled by the lack of published studies examining the effects of melamine and cyanuric acid in combination. One of these scientists, Birgit Puschner, a veterinary toxicologist at the University of California at Davis (UC Davis), explained: "We needed to determine with certainty whether or not melamine or cyanuric acid, alone or in combination, could cause renal disease."

To do this, she and her UC Davis colleagues performed three studies. They fed melamine alone, melamine and cyanuric acid in combination, and cyanuric acid alone, in various doses, to cats. To minimize the number of cats used in these studies, they did the experiments sequentially with just four animals. First, they gave melamine mixed into pet food to two cats; the cats survived and were used in the next experiment. In the second experiment, the UC Davis scientists fed melamine and cyanuric acid together to the two cats from the first study as well as to a third cat; each cat was fed a different dose. In the third experiment, the scientists fed cyanuric acid alone to the fourth cat, which had eaten only untainted pet food while serving as a control in the previous experiments. All of the cats were euthanized at the end of the studies so their tissues could be examined. The results of these experiments were reported in a conference call in September and published in a veterinary science journal in November. Similar experiments done on pigs at Iowa State, with similar results, also were reported in the September conference call, and P&G scientists were rumored to have obtained similar results in mice.

In the studies at UC Davis, the two cats fed melamine alone consumed doses ranging from 32 to 181 mg/kg. The cats did fine on all doses within that range; they showed no ill effects. This might be expected, as the highest dose, 181 mg/kg, is below the 250 mg/kg level that caused problems in some, but not all, sheep in the South African studies. The cat fed cyanuric acid alone also consumed doses ranging from 32 to 181 mg/kg, and it also did fine. This too would be expected from the sheep studies of the

1960s, in which investigators observed cyanuric acid to be safe even at doses 20 to 100 times higher.

The cats fed both chemicals, however, did not do well at all. Even at the lowest dose—32 mg/kg body weight for each chemical—the cats vomited and stopped eating. Within 36 hours, all three cats fed the two chemicals in combination had signs of impaired kidney function and were excreting crystals in their urine. On autopsy, the cats' kidney tubules were packed with crystals of complexes of melamine and cyanuric acid. Without question, this combination of chemicals disrupts normal kidney function. Mixed with cyanuric acid, a dose of melamine well below the level considered safe can cause kidney damage.

As is standard practice in studies involving animals, and as stated in the UC Davis paper, this study had been approved by the university's Animal Care and Use Committee and was conducted in compliance with the Animal Welfare Act, U.S. Public Health Service Policy on the Humane Care and Use of Laboratory Animals, and the Guide for Care and Use of Agriculture Animals in Agricultural Research and Teaching. Professor Puschner explained why it was important to do the study: "The data will make pet food ultimately safer because now we know what to look for. We had to make some sacrifices but I hope a large population of pets will benefit from it."

With the mystery of the toxic contaminant resolved at last, the next puzzle to solve was how melamine and cyanuric acid got into the wheat gluten in the first place. This meant tracing the melamine and cyanuric acid back to their origins in China.

13

....

THE CHINA CONNECTION

Menu Foods initially suspected that something might be wrong with the wheat gluten in its pet foods because the ingredient came from a new source. Menu had recently switched suppliers and in November 2006 began buying wheat gluten from Chem-Nutra. ChemNutra did not actually manufacture the ingredients it sold. It got them from China.

ChemNutra's very business is to import food and feed ingredients from China. The company explains on its website that its expertise is as "the China source experts." At the time of the recall, ChemNutra promised its clients "ultra-competitive" prices and the skills to "bridge the [Chinese] business and cultural gaps . . . including all regulatory, compliance, import and transportation requirements." ChemNutra made its living by making it easy for American companies to obtain Chinese food ingredients at prices much lower than those charged by American firms. At that time, Chinese wheat gluten cost 60 cents per

pound, an amount 20% to 30% lower than the cost of produc-
ing—let alone selling—this ingredient in the United States.

ChemNutra's Wheat Gluten

On March 8, Menu Foods told ChemNutra that something in
the wheat gluten might be causing cats to get sick. Since Chem-
Nutra did not actually manufacture this ingredient, the company had to discuss the matter with its supplier in China, the
Xuzhou Anying Biologic Technology Development Co., based
in Jiangsu. Xuzhou Anying's website, which was still active in
April 2007 (but has since disappeared), described its corporate
policy as "Sincere and Keeping Promise." Xuzhou Anying sold
wheat gluten under the title "Wheat Vital Protein." It also marketed something called "ESB Protein Powder," sold as a source
of non-protein nitrogen. Here is how Xuzhou Anying described
the ESB protein powder:

> Reasonably making use of NPN [non-protein nitrogen] and
> reducing the production cost of feed factor . . . After eating this,
> protein powder will be transformed into mycoprotein in the
> alimentary canal under the action of digestive enzyme; it will
> be normally digested, absorbed and used by the livestock and
> poultry. It is safe nonpoisonous, without bad reaction.

It is difficult to know how much of this description gets lost in
translation, but there are certainly some odd things about it.
Mycoproteins are fungal, not bacterial, proteins highly unlikely to
be produced by bacteria living in the stomachs of ruminant animals. In any case, non-protein nitrogen, no matter how "vital,"
cannot be used by poultry; chickens do not have rumens. It seems

likely that neither Xuzhou Anying's wheat gluten nor its ESB "protein" powder were made with protein but instead contained non-protein sources of nitrogen such as melamine or cyanuric acid. The most benign interpretation of the substitution is that the Chinese suppliers did not know that these chemicals could damage the kidneys of livestock and also did not know that chickens are incapable of converting non-protein nitrogen into protein.

A less benign interpretation, however, is that the company knew exactly what it was doing. David Barboza, a reporter for the *New York Times* stationed in Shanghai, found advertisements for melamine on the Xuzhou Anying website: "Our company buys large quantities of melamine scrap all year around." In fact, melamine was widely available for sale by Chinese suppliers. The website of one supplier, the Melamine Material Factory in Anhui, boasted that it was the largest manufacturer of this material in China.

At the end of March, when melamine was identified as the contaminant in wheat gluten, the FDA banned further imports of ingredients from Xuzhou Anying. This action set off a series of additional recalls by Hill's Pet Nutrition, Nestlé Purina PetCare, and Del Monte Pet Products, all of which were using Xuzhou Anying wheat gluten from ChemNutra. One of the Hill's products included a dry cat food, so this recall extended the range of affected products from wet to dry. On April 2, ChemNutra issued its own recall of the wheat gluten. This set off one more recall, this time by Sunshine Mills, which made pet foods with wheat gluten obtained from an intermediate supplier (Scoular) who got it from ChemNutra who got it "from a specific manufacturing facility in China." Figure 1 in Chapter 3 summarizes the connections among these events.

With so much at stake, relations between Menu Foods and ChemNutra lost all semblance of cordiality. In ChemNutra's version of the events:

> Menu Foods knew there was a potential problem long before we did . . . On or about March 6, Menu Foods informed us that it didn't want any more wheat gluten. They told us that it was because of a need for a different water absorption factor . . . On March 8 Menu Foods told us that our wheat gluten was one of many products it was investigating, so clearly they already had an investigation well in progress . . . The word "melamine" wasn't mentioned by anyone until late in the day on March 29, when the local FDA investigator returned to tell us he found melamine . . . All of our customers except Menu Foods understand that we were victims in this situation.

Victims? Perhaps not, as I will explain in Chapter 20.

But if the business about the "water absorption factor" is correct, Menu Foods must have been reluctant to admit that its foods might be causing problems and hopeful that it could delay taking action to correct them. ChemNutra also defended itself against charges that its customers did not know it was importing ingredients from China. ChemNutra said everyone knew its ingredients came from China, and posted photographs on its website to prove it. The photographs showed bags of wheat gluten clearly labeled "Made in China." A spokesperson for Chem-Nutra explained that the company was only a co-broker of the tainted wheat gluten: "We never owned it; we never sold it." And by implication, "We are not responsible for it."

The Menu Foods version of these events differs in some respects. For one thing, Paul Henderson, Menu's president and CEO, preferred to frame the crisis so it did not focus on his company. He referred to the events as the "Melamine and Related Compounds (MARC)" recall. For another, he said: "Unfortunately, we now know that ChemNutra provided Menu Foods and other pet food manufacturers with a product that was contaminated with melamine. Needless to say . . . we no longer do business with ChemNutra." Indeed, Menu filed a suit against ChemNutra, explaining that "ChemNutra's actions have caused tremendous injury to the public and to Menu." One can assume that the courts will eventually sort out who did what to whom, but none of this finger-pointing was of much use to grieving owners of dead pets or people desperate for truthful information about what was safe to feed their still healthy animals.

Denial of an Open Secret

Menu Foods, according to ChemNutra, merely asked it to find out from Xuzhou Anying whether the wheat gluten contained propylene glycol, heavy metals, or a toxin from the Easter lily, any of which might be a possible cause of kidney damage in cats. ChemNutra's CEO, Steve Miller, flew to China and personally met with the president of Xuzhou Anying on March 30 (the day after the FDA told him melamine had been found in the wheat gluten) to "demand more information." By ChemNutra's account, Xuzhou Anying's president "claimed no knowledge of how melamine contamination could have occurred and promised to investigate. Since then he has been unresponsive to requests for information . . . We are very distressed."

On April 2, the *New York Times* quoted Chinese officials denying that the country's exported ingredients were the cause of the pet deaths: "The poisoning of American pets has nothing to do with China." Xuzhou Anying officials continued to say they had no idea how melamine could have gotten into the wheat gluten and had nothing to do with the problem: "We are a trading company and don't manufacture the product." Instead, they explained, the wheat gluten came from 25 manufacturers in neighboring provinces. Weeks later, after much investigation, the FDA said it could not identify any of those manufacturers (if they existed at all) and concluded that the source of the melamine was unlikely ever to be determined. Xuzhou Anying's manager, Mao Lijun, repeatedly denied shipping wheat gluten to the United States but said the matter was under investigation.

When the *New York Times* reporter, David Barboza, visited Xuzhou Anying's main offices, he saw "just two rooms and an adjoining warehouse." A truck driver told him the company owned a factory that made wheat gluten but that the place was locked. Other Chinese producers of wheat gluten said they had never heard of anyone mixing it with melamine.

Barboza, however, must be an exceptionally persistent reporter. He found Chinese informants who were willing to talk to him about what had apparently been a wide-open practice. For years, they said, producers mixed melamine into feed for animals and fish. One informant told him: "It just saves money if you add melamine scrap." Another said: "No law or regulation says 'don't do it,' so everyone's doing it . . . If there's no accident, there won't be any regulation." And in a statement guaranteed to dismay any pet lover, a third told him: "If you add it [melamine] in small quantities, it won't hurt the animals . . . Pets are not like pigs or chickens . . . They don't need to grow as fast."

Barboza's conclusion from these revelations: "Melamine is the new scam of choice." The Chinese told him that they would much prefer to use urea, the chemical from which melamine is synthesized, as an adulterant. Urea is cheap and harmless as a source of non-protein nitrogen, but much too easy to detect. Companies used melamine because it was harder to detect and almost as cheap; real wheat gluten cost five times as much. Getting wheat gluten prices for melamine and its by-products was highly desirable. Chinese producers of animal feed told Barboza that they also liked using cyanuric acid "because it was cheaper and helped increase protein content." Adding cyanuric acid as an adulterant to fish meal, for example, would be cheaper than using melamine. From the standpoint of these suppliers, melamine and cyanuric acid were good nitrogen sources, were harmless, and made excellent business sense.

The Shipping Scam

But the revelations did not end there. Strictly speaking, Xuzhou Anying officials were telling the truth when they denied shipping adulterated wheat gluten to the United States. They did not actually do the shipping. Instead, they used another company as a cover—the wonderfully named Suzhou Textiles Silk Light Industrial Products Arts and Crafts Import and Export Company. By shipping through Suzhou Textiles, Xuzhou Anying could avoid having to register the adulterated wheat gluten as a food ingredient and subjecting it to inspection by Chinese food authorities. This creative approach to bypassing inspection first came to light when ChemNutra provided copies of a bill from Suzhou Textiles. The bill was for $18,920 for 24.3 tons of wheat gluten shipped on September 29, 2006. That wheat gluten, from an unnamed Chinese supplier, must have been the real thing, as it arrived two months earlier than the earliest date on which the recalled products were produced. As part of the standard pattern of denials, however, officials of Suzhou Textiles said they had not shipped wheat gluten to America. Later, the FDA's investigations of how all this occurred led a federal grand jury to issue indictments against officials of ChemNutra, Xuzhou Anying, and Suzhou Textiles for hiding the shipping of a tainted product from Chinese inspectors (see Chapter 20).

Suzhou Textiles, as it happens, runs a complicated business. Prior to the indictment, it maintained two active websites, both listing the same company name, manager (William Gu), and address (6 Xihuan Road, Suzhou). One site appeared to sell textiles: "Our company has dealt with import & export business for more than 15 years. We deal with many kinds of textiles and garments, including woven garments, knitwear, scarf etc." But a Google search also turned up an entirely different web address, this one explaining that Suzhou Textiles is in the business of exporting pharmaceutical raw materials such as food and feed additives, amino acids, chemicals, herb extracts, and, oddly, silk scarves:

> There are so many pharmaceutical and chemical manufacturers (more than 10 thousands) in China . . . Our task is to help our factories promoting their products in world market and help our customers . . . to achieve the lowest costs and efficient service . . . As a trading company and sales agent and sometimes broker, something we always keep in mind - quality & price, professionality & efficiency, reliability & reputation since we understand very well that "if we don't, someone else will."

That may be an accurate explanation of the company's management ethic, but melamine, cyanuric acid, and wheat gluten did not appear on Suzhou Textiles' long list of available pharmaceuticals. Even so, I was surprised that one company could export such a wide range of chemicals—and scarves—with such a small number of employees. Its company profile listed the number of "staffs" as fewer than five people and the number of workers also as fewer than five. More Google searching turned up yet a third site, last active in October 2007, listing the number of employees as 50 to 100. Taken together, the collective websites conveyed the uneasy impression that Suzhou Textiles was in the business of exporting pharmaceuticals under the guise of silk scarves.

One might think that these revelations were sufficient and it was time for this drama to come to a close. But no. This was merely the end of Act I.

14

....

MORE MELAMINE:
RICE AND CORN "PROTEINS"

In Act I, the distribution of melamine-laced wheat flour sold as wheat gluten began with unidentified manufacturers in China and ended with pet foods fed to cats and dogs in the United States. Complex as it is (see Chapter 3), the chain of distribution thus far turns out to be woefully incomplete. For Act II, we must return to early April and introduce yet another distributor of Chinese ingredients, the San Francisco–based Wilbur-Ellis Company. On April 4, Wilbur-Ellis found a bag labeled "melamine" in one of its shipments of another food ingredient imported from China, rice protein concentrate. This ingredient is similar to wheat gluten and is used for similar purposes. Wilbur-Ellis must not have paid much attention to this discovery because the company did not mention it for a couple of weeks.

Rice protein concentrate comes with its own convoluted chain of distribution, as shown in Figure 4. Wilbur-Ellis obtained the ingredient from a Chinese supplier, Binzhou Futian Biology Technology Co., in Shandong. Binzhou Futian, in turn, got the

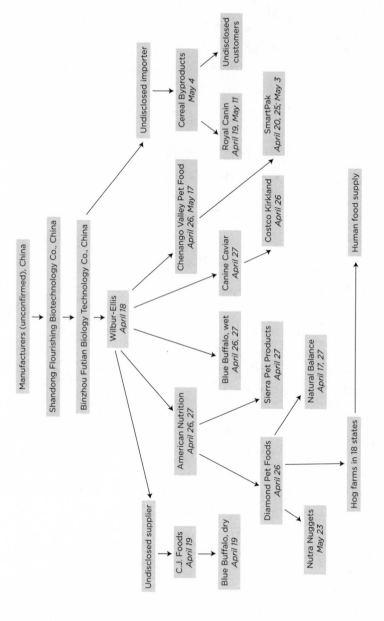

Figure 4. Partial chain of production and distribution of melamine in wheat flour sold as rice protein concentrate. Dates in italics indicate dates of recall notices. Companies are located in the United States unless otherwise indicated.

rice protein concentrate and a similar ingredient, corn gluten, from yet another company, Shandong Flourishing Biotechnology. A visit to the website of Shandong Flourishing in late April 2007 was a disconcerting experience. Here, for example, in direct quotation, is how Shandong Flourishing explained its management philosophy:

> Our company's management idea is: The good faith for this, by guaranteed the product quality strives for the survival, by creates the enterprise core competition to make every effort to develop, Persisted the user supreme principle, "thought the user thought, the anxious user is anxious". Our company seriously pledged to you that, Most superior quality! Most inexpensive price! Most arrives service! . . . Shandong luck Switzerland auspicious biotechnology limited company zealous welcome general new and old customers presence instruction, discussion service!

A description like this one readily explains why American companies would be grateful to be able to buy Chinese ingredients through experienced intermediaries such as ChemNutra and Wilbur-Ellis.

On the American side of the distribution chain, Wilbur-Ellis shipped the rice protein concentrate to several pet food manufacturers. Figure 4 outlines my best guess as to the chain of production and distribution of melamine-laced wheat flour unwittingly purchased by Wilbur-Ellis as rice protein concentrate.

On April 13 or close to it, Natural Balance Pet Foods heard four complaints that pets became ill after eating some of its products made with venison. Four or five more such complaints came in the next day. Frank Koch, the company's executive vice president, told me that Natural Balance had been so concerned about melamine that it had demanded—and received—a certificate from the Chinese supplier that the rice protein was free of that adulterant. Nevertheless, the company tested the products for melamine. Bingo. Natural Balance ordered a recall.

This recall must have reminded Wilbur-Ellis of the odd bag of melamine in its shipment from China. Wilbur-Ellis told the FDA about the bag and issued a recall of its rice protein concentrate. The supplier, Binzhou Futian, issued the usual denial of responsibility. Its officials told Wilbur-Ellis that "the contamination occurred through accidental reuse of dirty packaging."

Later analysis showed that the rice protein concentrate had nothing to do with rice. It turned out to be precisely the same adulterated product that had been imported by ChemNutra— wheat flour containing cyanuric acid as well as melamine. But the discovery of melamine in what was purported to be rice protein concentrate set off another flurry of recalls. One of these recalls included a dry food for ferrets made by Chenango Valley— another extension of the reach of the tainted ingredients. Some of the rice protein concentrate recalls deserve additional comments.

Royal Canin's Recall

Royal Canin, for example, recalled a group of dry dog foods ostensibly containing rice protein concentrate on April 19. The company (owned by Mars Petcare since 2001) obtained the ingredient from a firm in Illinois, Cereal Byproducts, which in turn obtained it from Binzhou Futian through yet another company identified only as a "domestic importer." On May 4, Cereal Byproducts issued its own recall of rice protein concentrate, which it said had been shipped to three midwestern customers as early as July 19, 2006—pushing the date of suspect products back even further into 2006. As is typical, "Cereal Byproducts assures its customers that the safety and quality of the ingredients it supplies is a top priority."

Royal Canin had to deal with yet another melamine-contaminated ingredient in its products—corn gluten. The company used corn gluten as an ingredient in pet foods manufactured in South Africa and Namibia, and the recall affected products made between March 8 and April 11, 2007. At least 19 dogs in Cape Town and Johannesburg fed Royal Canin Vets Choice foods had been diagnosed with acute kidney failure. But, said the company, its African customers "can rest assured that Royal Canin remains committed to putting the interests of pets and their health and nutrition first."

In repeatedly quoting such statements of assurance, I do not mean to suggest that pet food companies were necessarily insincere in their sentiments. But their words and actions suggested that the companies had little knowledge of where the ingredients in their products came from or what the ingredients contained.

Blue Buffalo's Accusations

The travails of Blue Buffalo are especially poignant. This company markets expensive "healthy and holistic natural foods for dogs and cats" directly to "pet parents." Within a week of the first recalls, Blue Buffalo ran a full-page ad in *USA Today:* "You love them like family. So feed them like family. Most pet foods contain animal by-products and things you'd never feed your family—but Blue is true." The ad provided a checklist: "no wheat gluten, no animal byproducts, no corn or soy protein."

The checklist did not include rice protein. Once Blue Buffalo learned about melamine in the rice protein concentrate, the company issued recalls on April 19, 26, and 27. By the last of these recalls, Blue Buffalo had withdrawn one-third of its product lines from sale.

According to *USA Today,* Blue Buffalo said it did not know that its rice protein concentrate came from China. In this instance, I can easily understand why. Blue Buffalo's dry and wet foods are manufactured through separate supply chains. Its dry cat foods are made by C.J. Foods ("pet food extrusion experts" in Pawnee City, Nebraska). C.J. Foods bought the rice protein ingredient from an unnamed supplier who, in turn, bought it from Wilbur-Ellis.

Blue Buffalo's wet dog and cat foods, however, were made by American Nutrition (Ogden, Utah), a company like Menu Foods. Blue Buffalo's recipes for its wet products did not specify rice protein concentrate as an ingredient. In the general framework of finger-pointing typical of these events, Blue Buffalo titled its April 26 recall notice "Blue Buffalo recalls can and biscuit products due to tampering by American Nutrition Inc.":

> American Nutrition Inc. (ANI), the manufacturer of all our cans and biscuits, has been adding rice protein concentrate to our can formulas without our knowledge and without our approval . . . It appears that only an FDA investigation of ANI's rice protein concentrate supplies forced them to reveal this product tampering to us . . . And while we test for known toxins and contaminants, we don't test for protein sources . . . especially when we did not formulate our products to contain them. In the end, this all comes down to an issue of integrity, and ANI has not been honest with us and with the pet parents who buy our products.

Diamond Pet Foods and Sierra Pet Products (Harmony Farms brands) also issued press releases saying that their products had not been formulated or labeled to include rice protein concentrate. This constituted a "manufacturing deviation." American Nutrition, they said, put rice protein concentrate in their products without their knowledge or consent.

American Nutrition's Rebuttal

To answer such charges, American Nutrition issued its own press release, remarkable for pointing fingers not only at its supplier, but also at its customers:

> American Nutrition did not engage in any deliberate or intentionally wrongful conduct . . . Rice protein is an ingredient commonly used in pet products to fortify protein content and provide proper texture and consistency of canned pet products . . . rice protein shipped from Wilbur-Ellis to American Nutrition was found to contain concentrations of melamine . . . products affected by the contaminated rice protein recall had customer-driven formula specifications for non-soy, non-corn, and non-wheat ingredients . . . customers specifically required rice-based formulations . . . Our utmost concern is for the health of the pets that consume our products.

I can understand why all of these companies were upset. If American Nutrition added rice protein concentrate to the product formulas and did not list the ingredient on the label, the FDA would consider the products to be misbranded and the companies would be subject to "enforcement," meaning product seizures, injunctions, and other unpleasant legal matters. If the companies really did not know about the switch in ingredients, I am guessing that American Nutrition did not think the substitution would matter for pet foods. If so, this would be a serious misreading of its customer base. Pet owners want more information about what is in the foods they are feeding their animals, not less, and precisely because they worry that manufacturers will make whatever substitutions they please and assume such switches will go unnoticed.

Acts I and II had moments of comedy and tragedy, but the drama was mostly restricted to the food supply for pets. Act III extends the chain of distribution of the tainted ingredients into broader areas of the food supply, this time into foods for farm animals and fish and, therefore, into foods that humans might eat.

15

....

MORE MELAMINE EATERS:
FARM ANIMALS AND PEOPLE

Following the trail of distribution of the fraudulent wheat gluten and rice protein concentrate is complicated by the ubiquity of
these ingredients in human foods. Protein ingredients are used
as thickening and coloring agents in foods as diverse as baby
foods, breads, cereals, pizza dough, mustards, soy sauce, malt
vinegar, protein shakes, energy bars, salad dressings, and soup
mixes. So an important reason—perhaps the main reason—the
FDA devoted time and resources to the pet food recalls was to
prevent whatever was causing kidney failure in cats and dogs
from getting into the human food supply.

As then Assistant FDA Commissioner David Acheson told reporters in the agency's teleconference on May 3, the FDA tested 700
samples of pet foods and ingredients and found melamine in 394 of
them (56%). All of the melamine-spiked ingredients had come
from just two Chinese importers, Xuzhou Anying and Binzhou
Futian. The FDA's investigations, however, found no evidence that
the contaminated ingredients had entered the human food supply:

Once we knew that the contaminated wheat gluten had ended up in the pet food supply, the obvious question was, had any of those contaminated lots gone down the human side of the arm? Had they gone into the human chain? We have done extensive investigations and follow up tracing forward and tracing back into that system and have found no evidence that any of those contaminated lots have ended up in the human food chain as an ingredient in human food.

But there was another route by which melamine could get into human foods, this one an especially unpleasant surprise—through farm animals that had eaten contaminated pet food. How melamine-tainted pet foods ended up in feed for animals that humans might have for dinner emerged in a series of revelations, one following right after another from mid-April to late May.

Food Animal Revelation #1: Pig Feed

On April 19, California state agriculture officials quarantined animals produced by American Hog Farm in the town of Ceres. The farm had fed salvaged pet food to its pigs, and laboratory tests identified melamine in their urine. American Hog Farm bought the salvage from Diamond Pet Foods on April 3 and 13. Diamond is the maker of the Natural Balance products that were recalled on April 17 because they contained melamine-laced wheat flour posing as rice protein concentrate. Diamond also sold salvaged pet food to hog farmers in five other states; these farmers also fed their animals without knowing that the pet food contained false rice protein concentrate contaminated with melamine.

I am willing to hazard a guess that I am not the only person who had no idea that farmers routinely feed salvaged pet food to pigs. I did not realize how tightly the pet, farm animal, and human food chains are interconnected. But given a moment's thought, feeding leftover pet food to pigs makes perfect sense. Pet food is highly nutritious and farmers are always looking for inexpensive ways to feed their animals. Pet food makers tell me that they are often approached by hog farmers eager to help with the disposal of discarded products.

By the time this part of the distribution chain came to light, farmers in six states had fed pet food tainted with melamine to about 6,000 pigs. Some of the pigs had already been sold to customers or slaughtering plants. One such plant, in Half Moon Bay, California, obtained 42 pigs from American Hog Farm and sold the meat to about 50 customers, some of whom owned restaurants. Most of the meat had already been eaten. So, melamine was now in the human food supply.

FDA officials were careful to explain that the hog farms had purchased damaged—not recalled—pet foods. In the FDA teleconference on April 24, Stephen Sundlof, then director of the Center for Veterinary Medicine, explained that selling salvaged pet food to pig farms was routine. Salvaged food was "someway damaged such that it can't be sold for pet food. It does not meet their quality standards or what have you. They often times sell that product to the livestock manufacturers." At the same teleconference, Captain David Elder, director of the FDA's Office of Enforcement, emphasized this point:

> These firms that shipped the salvage products to the hog farms
> did not do so after learning that their products were contami-
> nated. It is part of the routine business that salvaged and scrapped
> products that result from production [are] sent to farms like hog
> farms. So these weren't recalled products that were turned into

animal feeds . . . It was just part of the routine process and none
of that continued now that the contamination is known.

Because the U.S. Department of Agriculture (USDA) is in
charge of regulating meat and poultry production, this new development involved that agency as well as the FDA. On April 26,
the two agencies jointly announced that meat from 345 affected
hogs had entered the food supply. The remaining hogs would
be quarantined, and farmers would be compensated for their
losses. Officials insisted that meat from pigs eating melamine-
contaminated pet food had an extremely small chance of making
anyone sick. Why? Because of the "dilution factor." Melamine,
they said, would be so diluted by the time it got to human food
that its amount would be too low to be harmful. Melamine was
only a small part of rice protein; rice protein was only a small part
of pet food; pet food was only a small part of pigs' diets; and pork
is only a small part of the human diet.

With the food supply so seemingly out of control, this analysis—reasonable as it surely was—seemed less than reassuring.
The incident raised another troubling question: if the pet food
fed to pigs did not include products that had been recalled, where
were the recalled products? Captain Elder addressed this concern on April 24 in response to a question from a reporter:

> The disposition of the recalled material is going to be an obliga-
> tion of the recalling firm pulling it back and ensuring that it
> does not re-enter any type of food supply, human or animal.
> And they will need to dispose of it in accordance with State and
> Federal Environmental Laws. A possible way of doing so could
> be at a landfill or could be by incineration, but the recalling firm
> will ensure that the disposition is done appropriately and FDA
> will witness the disposition to make sure that nothing gets back
> out there into the food supply.

Steve Miller, ChemNutra's CEO, discussed the disposal problem during the congressional hearings on April 24. He said the contaminated wheat gluten had been quarantined in a warehouse. Later, as the class-action lawsuits progressed, it became apparent that ChemNutra wheat gluten was not the only substance under quarantine. The courts had impounded the pet foods recalled by companies involved in the litigation. By November 2007, companies were begging the courts for permission to dispose of the quarantined products. Del Monte Foods, for example, complained that it was storing 116,000 cases of recalled foods in warehouses in three states at a cost of $27,000 per month. Some of the products had been collected haphazardly and dumped into the equivalent of "banana boxes," where they had developed cracks and leaks. Del Monte submitted graphic photographs of vermin-infested containers in support of its pleas to destroy this key evidence.

But let's return to April, when ChemNutra was still working with the FDA to figure out what to do with the stored wheat gluten. As I discuss in a later chapter, the staffing situation at the FDA was such that it stretches credulity to think that the agency would be dropping everything else it was doing at that moment to supervise the disposal or even warehousing of 60 million cans and pouches of recalled pet food. Credulity was particularly stretched because salvaged pet foods were not just fed to hogs. They also were fed to chickens.

Food Animal Revelation #2: Chicken Feed

On April 30, the FDA and the USDA announced a second unpleasant surprise. Chicken farmers on about 30 broiler farms and eight breeder farms in Indiana had fed salvaged pet food (of unknown or undisclosed origin), this time containing melamine-tainted wheat flour in the guise of wheat gluten, to their flocks. This meant that 2.7 million broiler chickens consuming this food had already been processed, sold, and, no doubt, eaten. The two agencies asked owners of the remaining chickens—estimated at a not insignificant 100,000 breeder chickens—to euthanize them, and again promised compensation. They repeated the reassurance about melamine dilution. Nobody, they said, eats only chicken.

In reassuring the public about the safety of pigs and chickens that had eaten melamine, the agencies continued to insist that this chemical is not very toxic. They based this argument on the results of the FDA's toxicology review discussed earlier, the one commissioned to assess the effects of melamine and its by-products on human health. Released the week after the chicken revelations, that report described the feeding studies on rats and mice, did not refer to the studies on sheep and cattle, and said little about the role of cyanuric acid in reducing the level of melamine needed to induce crystal formation. The report concluded that neither melamine nor its by-products posed much risk to human health. In the May 3 teleconference conducted by the FDA, Dr. Acheson explained the connection between the distribution of the protein ingredients into separate food supplies for pets and people:

> I want to just clarify . . . to make sure that you all understand what I meant about pet food being used as human food. Well, I'm not trying to suggest that people are consuming pet food as part of a three-square meal. This is simply pet food that has gone through this pathway that I just alluded to in which it ended up in poultry and hogs, and therefore, wound up in the human food chain.

Food Animal Revelation #3: Fish

Surely chickens and hogs eating salvaged pet food would be the end of the story, but no such luck. A third unpleasant surprise arrived on May 8 when the FDA and the USDA jointly announced that melamine-laced wheat "gluten" had been shipped to a manufacturer of fish pellets in Canada in the summer of 2006. That company, Skretting, had then distributed the pellets to at least 60 hatcheries, pond-stocking facilities, and fish farms in Canada, and to nearly 200 such places in Washington State and Oregon.

FDA officials again reassured the public that the melamine-contaminated foods, in this case farmed fish, were safe to eat. Although the chickens were still being held, the FDA cleared the quarantined pigs for consumption. To demonstrate the extreme unlikelihood of harm coming to anyone eating meat from pigs that had eaten contaminated pet food, the FDA came up with a vivid example: "If you translate this into a 130-pound adult, they would have to eat more than 800 pounds of melamine-contaminated product in a day to reach that level. That—and if it was just the pork—it would have to be 800 pounds of pork." Unfortunately, the FDA did not explain how it arrived at this figure.

Food Animal Surprise #4: Melamine in Farm Feed

We are not done yet with this one. Difficult as it might be to imagine, a fourth unpleasant surprise—this one quite embarrassing—soon followed. It seems that the Chinese were not the only ones who were adding melamine to ingredients in farm feed.

Americans were doing this too. On May 18, Uniscope, Inc., of Johnstown, Colorado, a company that makes and distributes binding agents for animal feed, informed the FDA that it had found melamine in its products, some of which came from Tembec Inc., a company based in Toledo, Ohio. The melamine (from an undisclosed source) had been used to make feed for cattle, sheep, goats, fish, and shrimp.

The FDA began investigating the companies on May 21 but did not announce a recall until May 30. By that time, the companies had shipped the pellets not only to farms throughout the United States but also to farms in 13 other countries. The *New York Times* quoted the FDA's David Acheson as saying, "It's hard to believe that a manufacturer of pet food would not know about this." He must have meant animal feed—the binders were not in pet foods—but his annoyance seems entirely justified. Melamine is not approved as a feed ingredient and is not supposed to be used in animal or fish feed as a binder or for any other purpose.

Although the amounts of melamine in livestock feed were low (less than 50 mg/kg), the amounts were 233 mg/kg and 465 mg/kg in the fish and shrimp feed, respectively. The FDA said these amounts would be unlikely to pose a risk to human health. Indeed, shrimp do not eat large volumes of food, but what if cyanuric acid turned up in the mix as well?

With or without cyanuric acid, the FDA was not likely to cut Tembec much slack. A subsequent inspection of its plant revealed other "deviations" from the provisions of the Food, Drug, and Cosmetic Act. The FDA considered the company's products to be adulterated under the terms of the act because they contained unapproved food additives—melamine, among others. The

FDA also considered the products to be misbranded because the ingredient lists on the labels did not disclose the presence of melamine (having it there is one problem; not labeling it is another). As late as September, the FDA was still warning Tembec that the deviations had to be corrected or the company would face regulatory actions. To get out from under this threat, Tembec said it would no longer manufacture products regulated by the FDA. Fine, but the FDA wanted written confirmation that Tembec would stop making things it wasn't supposed to.

By the time these events unfolded, it was evident that the chains of production and distribution of food and feed ingredients were so deeply intertwined that a food getting into one part of the system had an excellent chance of getting recycled into other parts of the system. Pet foods have always been made from the leftover parts of slaughtered farm animals that are not going to be used for human food—the bones, organs, ears, and other nutritious by-products. The need for an outlet for the leftovers of animal slaughter is one of the reasons commercial pet foods exist. We now know the fate of salvaged pet food; it gets turned into feed for pigs, poultry, and farmed fish. I cannot resist having this unsettling thought: if federal officials had ordered the destruction of the pigs, chickens, and fish fed salvaged pet food, would their meat have been recycled back into pet food?

Never mind. Let's take a look at how the FDA handled its responsibilities in this crisis.

16

....

THE FDA'S RESPONSE

How the FDA handled the pet food recalls must be understood in the context of its limited resources and consequent need to prioritize, issues that I discuss in greater detail in Chapter 19. From the FDA's standpoint, its staff did everything possible to ensure public trust. At a meeting in November, Robert Brackett, then director of the Center for Food Safety and Applied Nutrition, said something like this (a paraphrase based on my notes):

> The FDA was stunned by the consumer response. Usually FDA consumer hotlines get 20 calls a day. This was hundreds or thousands a day. The FDA was honest and open, and that helped a lot. The FDA acted quickly. Pet food companies did not. The pet food crisis could have brought down the whole food safety system in the United States.

Figure 5 illustrates the FDA's approach to dealing with the pet food crisis. The FDA said that it had mobilized more than 400 employees in 20 district offices to take calls, conduct inspections

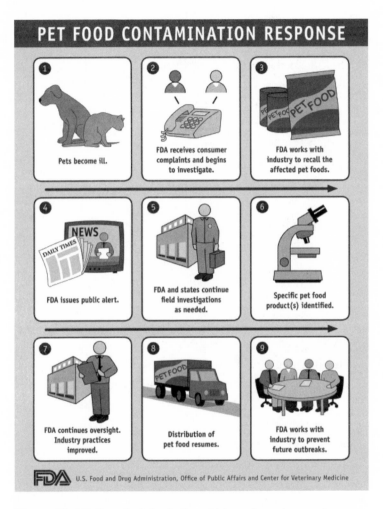

Figure 5. The FDA's methods for dealing with hazardous substances in pet foods. Source: FDA, www.fda.gov/cvm/petfoods.htm#PetFoodContamination.

and investigations, collect pet food samples, trace the source of the wheat gluten, and take care of the other matters illustrated in the figure. At the meeting in November at which I heard him speak, I asked Brackett about the 400 employees. He looked surprised and guessed they must have been part time.

A better idea of FDA staffing came in November in a report from the FDA's Science Board, a group appointed to advise the commissioner about scientific matters. The board noted that the pet food crisis had stretched the Center for Veterinary Medicine (CVM), the unit within the FDA that oversees pet foods and farm feed, far beyond its capacity. The CVM, the board observed, only had *two* full-time people working on pet food issues. The report did not say who these people were or what they were assigned to do, although it noted that 18,000 telephone calls came in about the recall.

With 18,000 calls and only two full-time staffers, FDA officials were confronted with a situation that would have overwhelmed any agency. Let's give them credit for organizing their first telephone conference with reporters within three days of Menu Foods' March 16 announcement and for holding such conferences every few days through the end of May.

Because the teleconferences were restricted to an hour or less, the transcripts sometimes make painful reading. The exchanges must have been frustrating for everyone concerned. Reporters were held in a telephone queue and were lucky if they could squeeze in a single question. Elizabeth Weise of *USA Today*, a frequent participant in these sessions, expressed some of this frustration during the teleconference on May 10 when she commented, "And having now become a connoisseur of these [teleconferences], I really like the new music they are playing for the hold music. Thank you." (The transcript does not note whether anyone laughed at her remark.)

Despite the restrictions and awkward format, reporters persisted in probing three key issues: the identity of the pet food manufacturers involved in the recall, the number of pets affected, and the potential harm of melamine to pets and people. In responding to questions about these matters, FDA officials often appeared to be uncertain of the facts, to be withholding critical information, or to be overly protective of the corporate interests of food companies.

Some of these problems may simply have been due to lack of information or communication within the agency. At the first teleconference on March 19, for example, a reporter asked Stephen Sundlof, the director of the CVM, to identify the company that had supplied the wheat gluten to Menu Foods. Mr. Sundlof replied, "I don't know what the name of the supplier is at this time." Let's assume he really did not know, but March 19 was the very day on which FDA investigators visited the headquarters of ChemNutra to demand documents related to its wheat gluten imports. During a teleconference held the next day, a reporter asked directly: "Who is that broker?" Mr. Sundlof's response: "Right now, we're not releasing that information." Reporters continued to ask who the broker was at subsequent teleconferences, but the FDA did not reveal ChemNutra's role in supplying the wheat gluten until April 5.

Reporters also asked the FDA to disclose the names of the companies making or selling pet foods containing wheat gluten that might have been contaminated. Because the FDA cannot order recalls, its officials felt constrained about identifying companies that had not yet gone public with their own recalls. The

FDA's reluctance to reveal this information led to some testy exchanges. Here is one from the teleconference of March 30:

> REPORTER: You have a manufacturer who has the wheat gluten. You don't know if it's in. They haven't called a recall yet and you just tell people to go ahead and feed food that has not been recalled yet. You don't know if the melamine is causing the actual death of the animals. What is the pet owner to think about what to feed their pet and what the FDA is doing for them?
>
> FDA [edited and condensed]: This is an ongoing investigation. We're following every lead we can. And my sense is that we have most of it under control.

The FDA gave similar responses during the April 19 teleconference (these excerpts are also edited and condensed):

> REPORTER: I'm wondering, since there are four other companies that we don't know about yet and we don't know if they're going to recall products, what are you telling pet owners? And they— should they just stop buying pet food . . . What would you suggest?
>
> FDA: We're suggesting as before to check our website . . . As soon as we find out that a product is subject to recall, it will be on the website. And that's pretty much the information that we can offer the public at this time.
>
> REPORTER: You . . . know the other three companies and you're not sharing it? . . . Shouldn't consumers have that information now so we can use it in our decision making process?
>
> FDA: When we have complete information, we share what we know when we know it. We are not going to share information that is speculative, that's preliminary. We are sharing information that FDA can stand behind.

The FDA must have known the names of manufacturers that had received shipments of the tainted protein ingredients, so its withholding of this information gave the appearance of protect-ing companies at the expense of the health of pets. This impres-sion was also conveyed by the FDA's stance on the number of pet illnesses and deaths. On this point, FDA officials were quite explicit, as illustrated in this April 26 exchange:

> REPORTER: Do you have a total number of pets either killed or sustaining some sort of injury from the pet food contamination, what figures do you have confirmed at this point?
>
> FDA: What I've previously said I believe in respond *[sic]* to the Washington Post question was . . . maybe 17 or 18 that we have confirmed. But again, that's not our focus. Our focus is to remove product that was contaminated, contained either wheat gluten or rice concentrate from commerce so we don't involve other animals or get into other parts of the supply system.

As late as November, the FDA was still minimizing the number of pets affected. That month, I participated in an FDA teleconfer-ence called to discuss the agency's new Food Protection Plan with people who cover food safety issues on Internet blog sites (see Chap-ters 19 and 20). To explain why the FDA had decided to reach out to bloggers, Commissioner Andrew von Eschenbach mentioned that in March his agency had been informed about the death of a small number of pets involved in a feeding study (the one con-ducted by the testing company recruited by Menu Foods to find out whether pets preferred to eat its foods or those of competitors). In this study, Eschenbach said, some of the pets unexpectedly died. Perhaps the commissioner did not mean to imply that the feeding study was all there was to it, but his remarks gave that impression.

As I noted earlier, FDA officials never did fully explain how much melamine the pet foods contained. In the May 10 telecon-ference, an FDA official said:

Melamine alone in relatively low doses is not toxic, it's not problematic. But when you start mixing it with cyanuric acid and other related compounds, it does appear to more readily form crystals. And it may be that these two batches [referring to the wheat gluten and rice protein concentrate] were high in cyanuric acid and melamine as opposed to just melamine. I'm speculating. I don't know.

Why didn't the FDA know? Had its scientists not bothered to measure the amounts of the chemicals in the pet food? Were they unable to make such measurements for some reason? Or did the amounts vary so much that no conclusions could be drawn? FDA officials did not discuss such questions and did not give reporters much time or opportunity to pursue them.

In the meantime, the FDA was taking other actions. It continued to pursue its investigations of ChemNutra's suspicious methods for importing wheat gluten from China and, presumably, its investigations of other importers involved in the recall. In April, it negotiated an agreement with the Association of American Feed Control Officials (AAFCO), the voluntary group of state officials who define the ingredients of animal feed and, therefore, pet foods. Under this agreement, the FDA agreed to recognize AAFCO definitions in return for the right to oversee any changes in ingredient formulations and to conduct scientific reviews of petitions for new ingredients. This agreement, which gave the FDA more control over the contents of animal feed, went into effect at the end of August.

To deal with the immediate problem of ingredients made in China, the FDA blocked imports of wheat gluten from Xuzhou Anying on April 3 and announced detention of all food ingredients from China on April 27. It set up a new website devoted to the melamine recall. The site listed the names of the companies issuing their own recalls but did not mention the names of pet food companies that were *not* voluntarily recalling their products. The FDA also steered clear of giving advice to pet owners or evaluating the extent of harm to pet health, explicitly leaving that task to veterinarians and bloggers. In May, the FDA issued a blanket warning to manufacturers reminding them "of their legal responsibility to ensure that all ingredients used in their products are safe for human consumption." None of this did much to encourage pet owners' confidence in the government's ability to protect their animals from unsafe food or, for that matter, to protect the safety of the food that they themselves eat.

To summarize the saga thus far, we have observed how the recalls exposed:

- the hazards of centralized manufacturing practices
- the difficulty of tracing the origin of food ingredients, especially those that are imported
- the weaknesses in oversight of food ingredients by food companies and by government
- the inextricable connections among the food supplies for people, farm animals, and pets
- the inadequacies of the FDA's ability to regulate the safety of pet foods
- the priority given to the interests of pet food companies at the expense of pet health

This last issue came up once again as the first anniversary of the recall approached in March 2008. The intrepid *USA Today* reporters discovered that scientists from Mars Petcare had known for a year that the Asian outbreak of pet kidney failure in 2004, which was caused by its Pedigree and Whiskas products (Chapter 12), looked the same as the outbreak caused by the foods recalled in 2007. Mars, Inc., a privately held company that is not required to disclose much about its holdings or operations, told the FDA about the link between the two outbreaks but made no public announcement. The FDA also said nothing. Why? Did FDA officials view the previous incident as irrelevant? Did they think nobody would be interested? Or were they protecting Mars? Late in March 2007, when Mars scientists made the connection between the two outbreaks, the company did not have products involved in the recalls. (Its recalls of Royal Canin products with rice protein concentrate came later.) Whether knowledge of the 2004 outbreak would have made any difference in the way the recalls were handled can never be known, but the nondisclosure appeared as further evidence of lack of concern for pets and their owners.

These problems with pet food companies and with the food system and its governance reflect some of the less desirable consequences of globalization. But along with their global causes, the pet food recalls had global repercussions. Let us now turn to some of those repercussions, beginning with the effects of the recall on food safety systems in the People's Republic of China.

17

....

REPERCUSSION #1:
CHINA'S FOOD SAFETY SYSTEM

China is so large in population and developing so rapidly that keeping up with events in that country is a formidable undertaking. But anyone who knows anything about the history of food safety in the United States will recognize what is happening with food safety in China. In the light of history, the fraudulent addition of melamine to wheat flour is neither unusual nor shocking. It is precisely the kind of fraud perpetrated by food producers in the United States in the heady years of booming commercial development prior to 1906. That year, of course, was the turning point in U.S. food safety regulation. In 1906, Upton Sinclair published *The Jungle,* his muckraking account of the horrors of the Chicago stockyards and meatpacking plants. His sensational account of those horrors appeared after decades of food adulteration scandals, but it caught public attention as none of those previous scandals had managed to do. Within a few months of its publication, Congress passed the Pure Food and Drug Act, which gave federal agencies the authority to create—and to enforce—

regulations designed to ensure the safety of the food supply. As Stephen Mihm explained in the *Boston Globe* in August, 2007:

> What's happening halfway around the world may be disturbing, even disgraceful, but it's hardly foreign. A century and a half ago, another fast-growing nation had a reputation for sacrificing standards to its pursuit of profit, and it was the United States ... Like China's poisonous pet-food makers, American factories turned out adulterated foods and willfully mislabeled products. Indeed, to see China today is to glimpse, in a distant mirror, the 19th-century American economy in all its corner-cutting fraudulent glory.

In passing off wheat flour as wheat gluten or rice protein concentrate, the Chinese were doing what unregulated food producers have always done: whatever they can get away with. Food regulations keep most food producers honest, especially when the regulations are thoughtfully designed and strictly enforced. In a country like China, in which food manufacturing is widely dispersed among untold numbers of small producers and regulations are nonexistent or just starting to be developed, an "anything goes" environment is only to be expected. It often takes a crisis to make governments realize that they need to take action. The pet food recalls were just such a crisis.

In the context of unregulated free enterprise, it is easy to understand why the first reactions of Chinese officials and company managers were, as one commentator put it, "petulant, passive-aggressive, [with] a lot of denial" of their responsibility for anything having to do with tainted ingredients. It is also understandable that when the FDA requested permission to go to China to investigate, Chinese officials might have wanted to postpone the intrusion until they could take care of the problems on their own. Indeed, the result was predictable. When the

Chinese finally relented and permitted FDA officials to visit, the Americans had nothing left to do. The Chinese had already closed down the two suppliers of the tainted protein ingredients and had arrested the managers of those companies.

China issued visas to FDA investigators on April 23. On April 24, Chinese officials sealed the premises of Binzhou Futian and forced the company to close. The next day, they detained Binzhou Futian's manager, Tian Feng, as well as the manager of Xuzhou Anying, Mao Lijun. In effect, these detentions were an admission that the companies had done something wrong. They also were a tacit admission that China's food safety system needed improvement.

China's Food Safety Problems

The pet food recalls focused worldwide attention on food safety problems in China. Although American consumers might have heard about safety incidents within China involving baby foods or foods contaminated with parasites, carcinogens, or banned drugs, these incidents seemed remote. The Chinese, however, were well aware of problems with their own food supply. One survey, for example, found 30% of American-branded foods sold in China to be counterfeit. Foods produced in China carried an unusually high risk of contamination because most of them— perhaps up to 80%—were made in small home kitchens or other sites with fewer than 10 workers. Hardly any of these small operations were licensed, as China did not have much in the way of food regulations, consumer protection laws, or inspection systems. The fraudulent wheat gluten and rice protein concentrate brought China's own problems with food safety into public scrutiny.

The Chinese government promptly announced that it intended to strengthen safety standards, increase inspections, require safety certifications, and tackle corruption in the food system and its oversight. Officials would be cracking down on the producers of unsafe foods. And they would be testing for toxins in cooking oil, flour, beverages, and baby foods. And so they did, big time.

In short order, China sent more than 33,000 inspectors into the field, conducted 10 million inspections, and shut down nearly 200 food manufacturers. Over the next few months, officials uncovered hundreds of thousands of food safety violations and closed down more than 150,000 unlicensed food businesses. The government said it would establish systems for food recalls, export inspections, and food safety standards, and would create a cabinet-level panel to oversee food safety and quality.

China's vice premier, Wu Yi, wrote that she herself held 10 national meetings on product safety and visited three provinces with a team of 300 inspectors. She reported that by the end of 2007, more than one million people in Guangdong alone had been trained in food safety procedures, and nearly all small food processing companies had "signed documents pledging food quality and safety." So let's give the pet food recalls some credit for improving food safety in China in the same way that *The Jungle* led to improvements in food safety oversight in the United States.

China has a huge population and its government acts on a grand scale. To prove to its own people and to the world that China would be taking its food safety problems seriously, officials arrested Zheng Xiaoyu, the former head of the state food and drug administration. They accused him of taking about $800,000 in bribes to approve drugs and put him on trial. On May 29, the courts sentenced him to death. Experienced China hands viewed this decision as an unusually clear signal that the government was committed to getting its food and drug safety problems under control. The courts also pronounced a death sentence on Cao Wenzhuang, another high-ranking food and drug official, but gave him a two-year reprieve. Zheng Xiaoyu was not so lucky. He was executed on July 10.

Later that month, Chinese officials revoked the licenses of Xuzhou Anying and Binzhou Futian and said they would pursue criminal proceedings against managers Mao Lijun and Tian Feng. For months, there was no word of these men. In February 2008, as I explain in Chapter 20, a federal grand jury in Missouri issued an indictment against Mao Lijun, along with officials of Suzhou Textiles and ChemNutra. On the day the indictment was announced, I sent an e-mail to David Barboza, the *New York Times* reporter in China, to ask if he had any idea what had happened to Mao Lijun and Tian Feng. Within an hour or so, I had his reply:

> Professor Nestle: Thanks for your email. I called Mao Lijun today and I believe he answered the phone—then denied he was Mao Lijun and hung up. It seems he's got his old email and is not in prison. I haven't heard about the other guy at Binzhou, but I'm going to try to find out.

No further news of them had arrived by the time this book went to press.

China's Trade Problems

Given the complicated supply chains, the sources of ingredients can be hard to trace and it is understandable that some pet food manufacturers were astonished to learn that their wheat gluten

or rice protein concentrate came from China. But their customers were even more astonished. Thus, the recalls revealed yet
another little known fact about the North American food system; many of our food ingredients—and our foods—come from
China. To give just a few examples from 2006 and 2007:

- *Food ingredients:* China was the largest supplier to U.S.
  companies of food additives such as vanilla flavoring,
  citric acid, and B vitamins. It made 60% or so of the
  world's supply of vitamin C. In 2006, China supplied
  14% of the wheat gluten used in the United States.
- *Fruit and vegetables:* China accounted for 50% or more
  of apple imports to the United States and for 12% of the
  global trade in fruits and vegetables. These are mostly
  processed products, but China was also a leading supplier of fresh garlic and mushrooms. Canada imported
  10 times as much fresh garlic from China in 2006 as it
  did in 2003.
- *Fish and seafood:* China was the largest supplier of farm-
  raised fish, both worldwide and to the United States. In
  2006, China supplied 21% of all U.S. seafood imports,
  80% of imported catfish and eel, and 12% of shrimp.
- *Animal food products:* China supplied 24% of the animal
  food products imported to the United States in 2006.
- *Animal feed:* Chinese exports of animal feed to the
  United States increased seven-fold from 2001 to 2006.
- *Pet food:* Chinese exports of pet food to Canada tripled
  in just three years, from $1.8 million (Canadian) in 2003
  to $5.8 million in 2006.

North American companies, of course, are happy to import
food ingredients from China because its prices are so low. Up to

now, China has been able to produce ingredients cheaply because its energy and labor costs have been well below those in Europe, Canada, or the United States, and its manufacturing practices have been subject to fewer and less stringent regulations.

Beyond foods and ingredients, the pet food recalls revealed what an extraordinarily important trading partner the People's Republic of China was—and is—to the United States. Back in 1978, just before we established diplomatic relations with that country, China ranked 57th in imports to the United States. But by 2006 China was our number two trading partner and was soon expected to be number one. In 1980, we imported $5 billion worth of goods from China; in 2006, we imported a whopping $343 billion.

Much of our trade deficit is owed to China. The last year in which the United States exported more goods to China than we imported from that country was 1980. Ten years later, we bought $10 billion more from China than we sold to it, but by 2007 the difference was nearly $240 billion, a deficit larger than that for any other trading partner. China accounts for a significant portion of our agricultural trade deficit as well. The U.S. Department of Agriculture claimed a $5.7 billion trade surplus in 2006, but that balance did not include fish and seafood. When these are added in, as shown in Table 6, the American agricultural trade deficit is $3.5 billion.

The large volume of foods coming in from China raises all kinds of questions about their safety—pesticides, heavy metals, mislabeled ingredients, possible adulteration—especially because imports from China accounted for a large proportion of FDA rejections of food shipments in 2006. But foods are not the only items to raise safety questions. Incidents in 2007 alone involved

Table 6. U.S. agricultural trade balance, 2006 (billions of $)

Commodity	Imports	Exports	Balance of Trade
Meat, dairy, fruit, vegetables, and other agricultural products except seafood	65.3	71.0	+5.7
Fish and seafood	13.4	4.2	-9.2
Total	78.7	75.2	-3.5

Sources: USDA. Latest U.S. agricultural trade data, updated November 9, 2007, at www.ers.usda.gov/data/fatus/monthlysummary.htm. National Oceanic and Atmospheric Administration. FishWatch—U.S. Seafood Facts, at www.nmfs .noaa.gov/fishwatch/trade_and_aquaculture.htm.

such widely diverse consumer products as toys, tires, toothpaste, and cough syrup, leading *Advertising Age* to headline an August 20 article on the topic "Is China turning into the land of tainted products?" So another consequence of the pet food recall was to turn the safety of food imported from China into a major issue in trade negotiations, not only in the United States and Canada but also in Europe.

The safety of pet foods is by no means the only trade issue that strains relations with China. High on the list is that country's failure to stop the export of unsafe foods and consumer products. But these issues add to the already contentious relations between the two countries over China's enormous trade surplus, its ongoing disputes with the World Trade Organization, and its floating, undervalued currency. This collection of issues, along with those having to do with pet food safety, induced Congress to urge the Bush administration to take a more aggressive stance to resolve trade disputes with China.

In late May, the United States asked China for data on that

country's procedures for testing and quarantining food ingredients and announced new import requirements. China would now be required to register firms that export foods to the United States. China retaliated. It refused U.S. shipments of Sun-Maid golden raisins, which it said were contaminated with bacteria and sulfur dioxide. The FDA re-retaliated. It blocked imports of Chinese farm-raised seafood said to be contaminated with heavy metals released into the environment from coal-fired power plants and other sources of industrial waste.

In the midst of all this diplomatic jockeying, some Chinese officials continued to minimize their country's safety problems and to argue that the business practices of their exporters were no different from those of businesses in the United States. Chinese officials blamed the media: "Some foreign media, especially those based in the U.S., have wantonly reported on so-called unsafe Chinese products. They are turning white to black . . . One company's problem doesn't make it a country's problem." Wei Xin, a press spokesperson for China, said, "Isolated cases should not be blown out of proportion to mislead the public into thinking that all food from China is unsafe . . . Our government asks countries that import our products to treat Chinese exports in a scientific and fair manner and work with us to address the issue." But in a rare admission, a senior regulator warned that food safety problems could cause disease and threaten social stability: "Especially in the countryside, the food safety situation is not optimistic."

In response to the exposure of its food safety problems, China continued to vacillate between denial and action. In July, it pledged to reform its oversight of consumer product safety and offered rewards to citizens who would report safety violations observed in food manufacture. Officials also recruited Ogilvy Public Relations to help manage international concerns about its safety practices. But in September, China reverted to blaming the United States for its problems. The FDA, Chinese officials said, should be doing a better job of holding companies accountable. It should be screening exports and banning the more flagrant violators. In late October, the Chinese admitted that only about 80% of foods and 70% of the country's restaurants had passed safety inspections. To address this problem, they had arrested nearly 800 people found to be violating product safety laws (the fate of these people remained unreported).

In November, China passed a draft food safety law to regulate domestic food production and processing, to establish systems for analyzing and monitoring food safety risks, and to improve inspection of food imports and exports. One month later, China instituted new safety standards for more than 100 categories of foods and drugs. In January 2008, the government announced the success of its food safety campaign: "The tasks of the rectification campaign have been fulfilled completely and its objectives have all been reached . . . The illegal practice of using non-food materials and or recycled food to produce and process food has been basically eliminated." Perhaps, but one month later yet another scandal, this time involving heparin made by unlicensed small producers, suggested that the country still had a lot more work to do. Even so, it seems reasonable to ask if the pet food scandal had anything to do with China's massive efforts to improve its food safety system. Eternal optimist that I am, I'd like to think it did.

18

....

REPERCUSSION #2:
THE CHINA BACKLASH

Back in the United States, the recalls stimulated a backlash against imported foods in general, and those imported from China especially. Congressman John Dingell (Democrat, Michigan) put it bluntly: "The country is awash in dangerous food coming in from China and other places." Treasury Secretary Henry Paulson, one of the chief negotiators of trade policy with China, said: "Right now product and food safety is the No. 1 issue." Some large companies, such as Mission Foods and Tyson Foods, announced bans on all Chinese ingredients in their products. To some observers, the bans sounded more like politics than reality, as companies would not be able to replace what they were getting from China at such a low cost. And, as we saw earlier (Chapters 3 and 14), the supply chains involve so many intermediates that end users can hardly be expected to know where their ingredients come from.

Nevertheless, labels proclaiming "China-free" or "100% U.S.-sourced" began appearing on consumer goods. As an indication of the extent of food-safety fears, athletes who planned to participate in the summer 2008 Olympic Games in Beijing were warned to bring their own toothpaste and food, and the U.S. Olympic Committee made arrangements to have most of the food for U.S. participants shipped in. In response to unspecified concerns on the part of consumers, Trader Joe's, the specialty grocery chain, said it would no longer import foods from China such as garlic, frozen spinach, ginger, and cooked soybeans.

In February 2008 I attended Global Pet Expo, an enormous pet product trade show at the San Diego convention center. Company after company exhibited pet foods in booths decorated with American flags and signs proclaiming "no ingredients from China." One exhibitor told me that his company now bought all its pet food ingredients from Europe. Nobody, he said, was buying anything from China except taurine, an amino acid required in the diet of cats, and this was only because no company in the United States made this substance. I spoke with several representatives of Chinese companies that export rawhide dog treats and asked them how they were faring in this "don't buy from China" climate. They told me they were doing what they could to demonstrate the safety of their products and were just waiting for the crisis to blow over.

Eat Local

Fears of the hazards of imported foods lent support to the burgeoning "locavore" movement, which encourages the buying and eating of foods grown within a few hundred miles of home. Locavores cite many reasons for their movement. Because local foods don't have to travel so far or long, they are fresher and taste better. They save some of the fuel costs of transportation. They also save on what ecologists call "food miles," a term that refers not only to the distance a food travels from production to consumption, but also to the full range of social and environmental costs of industrialized food production: the pollution of land and water, health problems among farm workers and neighbors, the depletion of world supplies of fuel oil, and the contribution of agriculture to climate change. Locally grown foods, ecologists say, are better for health and the environment. As a bonus, support for small local farmers also promotes the viability of rural communities.

The pet food recall added one more rationale to the locavore movement: locally grown foods are safer. Because they are produced on a smaller scale, they are likely to have fewer problems with contamination. And if they do become contaminated, the contaminants are likely to affect fewer people. By coincidence, on March 12, 2007—in the very week that Menu Foods announced its first recall—*Time* magazine ran a cover story on the advantages of locally grown foods: "Forget organic. Eat local."

Label Country of Origin

The origin of many foods can be a mystery, not least because labels do not have to disclose where the foods or ingredients come from. This omission is a story in itself. In 2002, Congress passed a law requiring Country of Origin Labeling (neatly referred to as COOL) for a motley collection of foods—pork, beef, lamb, fresh fruits, vegetables, and seafood. But then, under relentless pressure from the industries affected by the law, Congress delayed putting it into practice. At first Congress postponed implementation of COOL until 2006 for everything except fish and seafood. Later, it delayed implementation again, until 2008. Fish retailers, however, were required to use COOL labels beginning in 2004 (the fish industry must have less skilled lobbyists or weaker political clout). But as far as I could tell, after fish COOL went into effect, few fish sellers used such labels, and many still do not. No federal agency seems particularly concerned about enforcing COOL for fish.

From 2002 to 2007, food industry opposition to COOL was just about universal. Food trade associations complained about the burdens of tracking, record keeping, labeling, and general government interference. As I discuss in my book *What to Eat,* the Grocery Manufacturers of America (later renamed the Grocery Manufacturers Association), ever vigilant, called the 2002 legislation "a nasty, snarly beast of a bill." The strongest opposition, however, came from the meat industry, which argued that COOL would be expensive to implement but would produce no discernible benefit. The industry's principal objection was that producers would have to track where animals and meat products come from, an idea that meat groups have long resisted. What the meat and other food industries preferred was voluntary COOL—presumably so they could voluntarily avoid labeling the origin of their products.

A glance at almost any supermarket in 2007 showed that with few exceptions, voluntary COOL was not working. One such exception is the Whole Foods chain, which somehow manages to label where its foods come from with no apparent difficulty. But other voluntary efforts are less successful. In December 2007, one of my New York University colleagues handed me a packet of Snak Club Gummy Bear candies with this label: "Product of

U.S.A. or Mexico or Brazil or Czech Republic or China or Indonesia." Not much help, that one.

The pet food recall stimulated new interest in putting COOL into practice, not least so consumers could figure out whether foods were imported from China. By coincidence, 2007 was also the year in which the Farm Bill was up for renewal, and Congress soon attached COOL provisions to that legislation. In July, the House passed a bill requiring full implementation of mandatory COOL, adding goat meat to the list of foods that would need to be labeled. The Senate version of the bill added macadamia nuts. When Congress returned in 2008 for its second session, the final bill was still in play. That's politics for you.

Congress may have been dithering, but constituents quite clearly wanted COOL. In a poll conducted in August 2007, 88% of 4,500 adults said they favored mandatory COOL and 95% said consumers had a right to that information. A strong majority—70%—said they would be willing to pay more for food produced in the United States. In a survey conducted in October, 690 of 1,000 Americans said they routinely check food labels for country of origin, and 860 said they think Chinese food imports should be suspended until the foods meet American safety standards. The American public wants COOL; the food industry does not. The pet food recalls exposed the dispute over COOL as an unusually clear example of food politics in action.

Establish Stronger Rules for Import Safety

With such strong public interest in food origins and safety, even a reluctant government ought to be able to act. On July 18, 2007, the White House announced that it was appointing the Inter-

agency Working Group on Import Safety for the purpose of proposing policies to deal with unsafe imports from China and other
countries. In September, the group presented a "Strategic
Framework" for addressing the import problem. Its report
advised the president to shift away from a system of "snapshots"
at the border

> to a cost-effective, prevention-focused "video" model that identi-
> fies and targets those critical points in the import life cycle where
> the risk of unsafe products is greatest . . . Such a risk-based,
> prevention-focused model will help ensure that safety is built
> into products before they reach our borders. Import safety is
> a public-private responsibility . . . Supporting this model are
> six building blocks: 1) Advance a common vision, 2) Increase
> accountability, enforcement and deterrence, 3) Focus on risks
> over the life cycle of an imported product, 4) Build interoperable
> systems, 5) Foster a culture of collaboration, and 6) Promote
> technological innovation and new science.

I have no idea what this paragraph might mean in practice
and was no better off after reading the full report. But food
industry groups had no such problem. They caught on right
away that the Working Group's recommendations would be
giving them plenty of leeway. In an act of stunning irony, the
Grocery Manufacturers Association (GMA), a trade association
legendary for its opposition to government regulation, suddenly
began pleading with Congress to impose more oversight on the
food industry. Citing inadequate regulation of pet food and the
resulting loss of consumer trust as principal reasons for its change
of heart, the GMA urged Congress to give the FDA more power
to enforce safety rules through what it called "Four Pillars," or
programs, all of them *voluntary,* of course: (1) quality assurance

for importers, (2) expedited handling for low-risk importers, (3) improvement of food safety systems in foreign countries, and (4) focus of resources on high-risk imports. In proposing this scheme, the GMA was "trying to get ahead of the regulation curve" while the industry-friendly Bush administration was still in place. A GMA official said, "Recent events have exposed some weaknesses in the nation's food safety net . . . We're not sitting back and waiting for the government to inspect us to a safe food supply."

In November, the Working Group produced a 68-page plan of action based on its framework ideas. Hardly accidental is the plan's striking similarity to the GMA proposals. The plan lists 14 recommendations, most of them beginning with reassuring terms such as "create," "verify," "strengthen," "maximize," and "harmonize," and all of them voluntary. Here's one: "Complete a single-window interface for the intra-agency, interagency, and private-sector exchange of import data." You may understand what this means; I do not.

The Working Group also listed 50 steps to be taken to ensure import safety. Some of these are vague: "Improve U.S. liaison to foreign countries," for example. Others contain some good suggestions for safety standards, certification of exporters, and penalties. One would authorize the FDA to refuse to admit products if the agency is denied the right to inspect the plant where they are manufactured. Another would allow the FDA to order the destruction of medical products that had been refused entry. The surprise here is that the FDA does not already have the right to take such basic steps.

Another recommendation addressed the vexing question of recall authority. The Working Group almost, but not quite, proposed granting the FDA that right: "Authorize FDA to issue a mandatory recall of food products when voluntary recalls are not effective." The wording here suggests that the FDA would first have to attempt to negotiate a voluntary recall; only when that failed could the agency exert its authority. How long those negotiations had to continue, the Working Group did not say. It also did not say much about the need for new resources to carry out these new responsibilities. Instead, it advised federal agencies to prioritize, to reallocate existing resources, and to request "additional funding needs through the normal budget process"—not exactly a strong call to action.

On the international front, however, the Bush administration was making some progress. In December, the United States and China entered into "The Third China-U.S. Strategic Economic Dialogue" to discuss mutual concerns about product quality and food safety. As Wu Yi, China's vice premier, explained, this dialogue

> shows that the two governments are committed to protecting people's livelihood and consumers' rights, and that China and the U.S. are working together to meet new challenges posed by economic globalization . . . individual cases involving product quality and food safety ought to be handled for what they are, and one should resist the temptation to jump to sweeping conclusions about them. In particular, attempts to politicize these issues and use them to erect new trade barriers should be firmly opposed.

The dialogue was most successful in the area of food safety. The two countries actually signed an agreement that, according to the *Los Angeles Times,* "gives the U.S. government a larger role in the screening of exports in a bid to restore consumer confidence." China agreed to register its exporters, allow U.S. officials to inspect production facilities, and permit the FDA to open an inspection office in China. But the agreement covered only a limited number of foods—preserved foods, farm-raised fish, and pet food ingredients. From the standpoint of China, the agreement was meant to resolve the "disharmonious notes" that had impaired trade relations between the two countries. A skeptical former FDA official told the *Wall Street Journal,* "While the [pact] can be helpful, it cannot at this time in China's history solve the problem." Presumably, he meant that the agreement could not be adequately enforced given the enormous volume of products traded between the two countries.

Fix the Domestic Food Safety System

Food safety is a global problem and, as we have seen, imported ingredients quickly become dispersed throughout the domestic food supply. In its piecemeal approach to recommendations, the Working Group on Import Safety did not address import linkages to the domestic food safety system in the United States, nor did it say a word about the need for a major overhaul of the domestic system. These issues, no doubt, were outside its mandate. But many public health authorities have long believed that the problems of food safety oversight in the United States are so deeply entrenched that nothing short of a complete overhaul will fix the situation. Their solution: create a single food agency that combines and rationalizes the gamut of federal food safety functions, particularly those of the FDA and USDA.

The General Accounting Office (since 2004, the Government Accountability Office) has argued forcefully, if ineffectively, for a single food safety agency since the early 1990s. More recently, the idea has gained support from such varied stakeholders as food safety advocates, some members of Congress, and even some candidates for the 2008 presidential election. Why such an entity seems to be the only possible solution to the problem of food safety oversight brings us to the next repercussion of the pet food crisis—widespread recognition of the FDA's diminished regulatory capacity and of the urgent need to strengthen that capacity.

19

....

REPERCUSSION #3:
THE FDA IN CRISIS

If the FDA could not keep contaminated ingredients out of pet foods, was it capable of protecting the human food supply? William Hubbard, a former FDA official, could not have expressed the need to strengthen food safety oversight more clearly: "I do think this pet food thing has shown people, including people at the very highest levels of the administration, that something needs to be fixed. If this is not a wake-up call, then people are so asleep they are catatonic."

Indeed, "this pet food thing" publicly exposed what food safety experts have been saying for years. The FDA is in trouble. It no longer has the capacity to protect the food supply. It still operates under food and drug laws passed in 1906 and modified in 1938, when the food supply was very different than it is today. Robert Brackett, then director of the Center for Food Safety and Applied Nutrition (CFSAN), explained his agency's challenge at a meeting I attended in November. According to my notes, he said something like "Globalization has changed the way the

FDA has to function. The system was designed for whole foods brought in from a 50-mile radius. Now we have food products that may contain ingredients from 50 countries." Earlier he had said:

> The regulatory framework is designed for a production system of 30 to 40 years ago—we don't live in that world anymore . . . We have 60,000 to 80,000 facilities that we're responsible for in any given year [along with] explosive growth in the number of processors and the amount of imported foods . . . We have to get out of the 1950s paradigm.

That paradigm involved what we would now consider to be a locavore's paradise, with food safety outbreaks limited to families eating leftover turkey stuffing or deviled eggs at a picnic. The 1906 law, even as amended in 1938, was not designed to cope with today's industrialized, centralized food production system. In this system, one batch of spinach contaminated with *E. coli* O157:H7 can be responsible for sickening 200 people in 26 states ranging from Maine to Oregon. The disconnection between the current food system and the laws designed to govern it has led to a fundamentally irrational system of food safety oversight.

The pet food recalls illustrated several aspects of this irrationality. As we have seen, the FDA cannot order recalls of potentially harmful foods. And although the food supplies for pets, farm animals, and humans are impossible to keep separate, the FDA has distinctly separate units for regulating these foods, each under its own rules. At the FDA, CFSAN is in charge of foods for humans, but the Center for Veterinary Medicine (CVM) oversees foods for pets and feed for farm animals. And yet another agency, the USDA, with its own separate ways of doing things, is responsible for the safety of pigs, cattle, and chickens that are eaten by humans but eat feed regulated by the FDA. The results of this dispersal of functions are gaps in oversight that are in part responsible for the succession of food safety crises that occurred in 2006 and 2007—from *E. coli* O157:H7 in spinach and beef to melamine in pet food—and that seem to be getting worse with time. In February 2008, for example, the USDA announced the largest recall of ground beef in history: 143 million pounds. Each successive crisis provides further evidence of the need to fix the system. For many observers, myself among them, the most likely fix is to start from scratch, consolidate food safety functions within a single oversight agency, and give that agency enough legislative, personnel, and financial resources to do its work.

The FDA's Resource Crisis

Why a single food safety agency seems like the only viable solution is best explained by a few basic facts about the existing system. Food safety oversight is largely, but not exclusively, divided between two agencies, the FDA and the USDA. The USDA mostly oversees meat and poultry; the FDA mostly handles everything else, including pet food and animal feed. Although this division of responsibility means that the FDA is responsible for the safety of 80% of the food supply, it gets only 20% of the federal budget for this purpose. In contrast, the USDA gets 80% of the budget for 20% of the foods. This uneven distribution is the result of a little history and a lot of politics.

First the history: the FDA started out in 1906 as a unit within the USDA but was successively transferred from one agency to another until it ended up in what is now known as the Department of Health and Human Services. The FDA's funding, however, stayed behind, remaining under the authority of congressional agricultural—not health—committees. The politics follows from this history: agriculture committees support agriculture, not health, and routinely assign higher priority to the demands of the USDA. But food safety oversight within the FDA and the USDA is unequal in another way: the rank of their leaders within the federal hierarchy. The chief food safety official within the USDA is an assistant secretary; the highest official at USDA is the secretary, so an assistant secretary is rank two. At the FDA, however, the top food safety official is an assistant or associate commissioner who ranks four or below in the federal hierarchy; the job reports to the commissioner, who reports to the assistant secretary for health, who reports to the secretary of Health and Human Services. In the federal government, these rank distinctions matter greatly in terms of authority, power, and who gets to sit at the conference table.

More resources for the FDA certainly would help, but it is hard to know where to begin to assess the need. To speak only of food inspections: the United States currently imports about 80% of its seafood, 32% of its fruit and nuts, 13% of its vegetables, and 10% of its meats. In 2007, these foods arrived in 25,000 shipments a day from about 100 countries. The FDA was able to inspect only about 1% of these shipments, down from 8% in 1992. In contrast, the USDA is able to inspect 16% of the foods under its purview. By one assessment, the FDA has become so short-staffed that it would take the agency 1,900 years to inspect every foreign plant that exports food to the United States.

Why is the FDA losing resources? Besides its problems with

agricultural appropriations and lower-ranked leaders, I think two things are responsible: dietary supplements and cigarettes. Congress, under pressure from industries enraged at the FDA's attempts to regulate these substances as drugs, systematically reduced the FDA's resources at the same time as it greatly increased the agency's responsibilities. These actions crippled the FDA's ability to protect the food supply as well as to carry out its other mandated functions. The resulting disarray is best seen in the FDA's present inability to act quickly and decisively on questions about the safety of prescription drugs.

After September 11, 2001, it seemed possible that Congress would act to strengthen the nation's food safety system. But calls for creation of a single food safety agency were ignored in the rush to create the Department of Homeland Security. Still, Congress provided enough funding to double the FDA's inspection rate to 2%. But that auspicious moment did not last. In the years following 2001, Congress allowed the FDA's resources to dwindle and the number of inspectors to decline by 20%. The result: of 200,000 food products coming in from China in 2006, the FDA sampled less than 2%. China may be the high-risk exporter that dominates the pet food story, but it is not the only country selling potentially unsafe food and its record is by no means the worst. In 2006, China ranked third behind India and Mexico in the number of food shipments refused by the FDA.

The Science Board's Critique

The low inspection rate, it turns out, merely skims the surface of the FDA's problems. Late in November 2007, the FDA's Science Board, a committee that directly advises the commissioner (disclosure: I was a consumer representative to this board from 1998 to 2001), issued a scathing report on the agency's condition. The board's overall finding: "Science at the FDA is in a precarious position" as a result of staff shortages and the inability to recruit and retain scientific staff. The board judged CFSAN and CVM to be so badly in crisis that the "FDA does not have the capacity to ensure the safety of food for the nation."

How could it? In 2006, as the board pointed out, CFSAN alone was responsible for $417 billion worth of domestic food, $49 billion in imported foods, $60 billion in cosmetics, and $18 billion in dietary supplements, while CVM was responsible for the safety of food for 200 million pets and more than 10 billion food-producing animals, not to mention the work of 90,000 manufacturers.

The board noted that the FDA suffered from a two-decade trend of expanded responsibilities undermined by drastic reductions in resources. From 1988 to 2007, Congress enacted 123 statutes that increased the FDA's regulatory responsibilities, but the agency's funding did not keep up with inflation. CFSAN was particularly hard hit; it lost 15% of its staff despite new mandates to regulate supplements, food labels, allergens, and food security. As for CVM, as I noted earlier, the board said:

> The recent pet food safety crisis has strained this overtaxed system. CVM received more than 18,000 telephone calls concerning melamine pet food contamination. The pet food industry is a $15 to $20 billion a year business and largely falls within FDA's regulatory purview. It was estimated that about 1 percent of the total volume of pet food was involved with a potential economic impact of $200 million. CVM is able to devote only two people working full time on pet food issues.

As an advisory committee to the FDA commissioner, the board is hardly in a position to recommend removal of the agency's food safety functions to a new federal entity. Instead, it did the obvious and recommended more resources: "FDA can no longer fulfill its mission without substantial and sustained additional appropriations." These, the board said, would not be all that difficult to obtain: "Currently each American pays about a penny and a half a day for the FDA; an increase to three cents daily would not, in our view, be a great price to pay for the assurance that our food and drug supply is, indeed, the best and safest in the world."

In reviewing the FDA's weakened scientific and technical capability, the Science Board left one other problem unmentioned, this one the elephant in the room: the political nature of the agency's leadership. The FDA's failure to maintain its capacity as a public health regulatory agency and to fight hard for the resources to do so must be understood in the context of its position as a unit within the Public Health Service (PHS), a subagency of the Department of Health and Human Services (HHS). Like the USDA, HHS is part of the executive branch of government. Higher officials of HHS, PHS, and the FDA are politically appointed, meaning that their jobs are to carry out the policies of whatever administration is in power. In this instance, the president was George W. Bush, a Republican with an especially industry-friendly outlook on the role of government. As some commentators have noted, Bush political appointees "operate with a single-minded focus that makes them very present in the day-to-day operation of the agencies, all the way down to the field levels." Political appointees, of course, are also responsible for appointing permanent FDA staff. In this environment, the FDA was not likely to ask for anything of which the White

House might disapprove. Given the politics, the Science Board's demand for more resources for the FDA took real courage.

The FDA's Food Protection Plan

The highly political nature of FDA leadership also explains some of the problems with its November 2007 strategic plan for food protection. The plan arrived in what was certainly a busy month for the FDA's political appointees in the policy and communications arenas. In November, the FDA's Science Board submitted its critique, and the president's Interagency Working Group on Import Safety issued its action plan (discussed in the previous chapter). On the same day the Working Group released its report, the FDA issued its Food Protection Plan, aimed at improving import safety. While all of these reports were pouring in, Robert Brackett, the director of CFSAN, announced that he would be leaving the FDA to join the Grocery Manufacturers Association as senior vice president and chief science and regulatory affairs officer, thereby becoming one of the legions of FDA officials who have passed through the revolving door between government agencies and the industries they regulate.

Designed to address the safety needs of a global food supply, the FDA's Food Protection Plan involved three elements: "Prevent, Intervene, Respond." It focused on high-risk foods and reliance on third parties—companies and foreign governments—to ensure that imported foods are safe. Even recommendations this mild required an extension of the FDA's current authority, meaning that they could not be accomplished without new congressional legislation. Table 7 lists the "Prevent, Intervene, Respond" elements of the plan that require new laws. What is most striking about this list is

Table 7. Elements of the FDA's 2007 Food Protection Plan requiring new legislation

Prevent Foodborne Contamination

- Allow FDA to require preventive controls to prevent intentional adulteration by terrorists or criminals at points of high vulnerability in the food chain.
- Authorize FDA to issue additional preventive controls for high-risk foods.
- Require food facilities to renew their FDA registrations every two years, and allow FDA to modify the registration categories.

Intervene at Critical Points in the Food Supply Chain

- Authorize FDA to accredit highly qualified third parties for voluntary food inspections.
- Require new reinspection fee from facilities that fail to meet current Good Manufacturing Practices.
- Authorize FDA to require electronic import certificates.
- Require new food and animal feed export certification fee.
- Provide parity between domestic and imported foods if inspection access is denied.

Respond Rapidly to Minimize Harm

- Empower FDA to issue a mandatory recall of food products when voluntary recalls are not effective.
- Give FDA enhanced access to food records during emergencies.

Source: FDA. Food Protection Plan: An Integrated Strategy for Protecting the Nation's Food Supply, November 2007, at www.fda.gov/oc/initiatives/advance/food/plan.pdf.

how fundamental some of the steps seem to be. The FDA was not already authorized to do those things? No, it was not.

On November 14, I participated in an FDA teleconference on the Food Protection Plan and was able to ask Commissioner Andrew von Eschenbach, most definitely a political appointee, how he expected to fund the new responsibilities. He replied that the FDA would be asking for resources in the 2009 budgetary process: "We are cognizant and they are built in." By this he meant that the FDA was aware of its resource needs and was requesting resources in the next budget cycle. Perhaps so, but asking is not the same as receiving, needing new legislation is not the same as getting it passed, and 2009 was not then due to arrive for another fourteen months.

I was by no means the only one concerned about weaknesses in the plan. Early in December, Congress held hearings at which food safety experts criticized the plan's focus on high-risk products. This focus, critics said, would not work because it required the FDA to wait until foods caused harm before designating them as high risk. Even the Grocery Manufacturers Association agreed that *all* imported foods should be expected to meet FDA safety standards, regardless of risk level. The influence of politics on the FDA's budget requests and proposed actions could not have been more evident.

The Confidence Crisis:
Another Mad Cow Catastrophe?

In reflecting on the pet food and other food safety crises of 2006 and 2007 a few months before he left his position as director of CFSAN, Robert Brackett said:

> The pet food scandal has the potential to become to the US food
> system what BSE was to the Europeans . . . One of the lessons
> from BSE in Europe was to be fully open and forthcoming
> about everything that was known—the key is to maintain the
> public's confidence in the system, and the best way to do so is to
> communicate openly, widely, and quickly.

As I mentioned in Chapter 16, Brackett also said that the pet food crisis could have brought down the country's entire food safety system. In that statement and the one about "BSE in Europe" he was referring to the crisis in Great Britain caused by the epidemic of bovine spongiform encephalopathy (BSE), better known as mad cow disease, in the early 1990s. The cost of this crisis—in money, lives, and livelihoods—was enormous. Five million cows were destroyed. More than 150 people lost their lives to the human variant of BSE as a result of eating meat from cows with the disease. Even pets were at risk; the British reported 89 deaths among cats eating pet foods made from by-products of cows sick with BSE.

One additional unhappy consequence of the mad cow crisis was the loss of public trust in the British food industry and its government regulators. In a series of infamous incidents, government officials denied both the extent of the illness in cows and the possibility that the disease could be transmitted to people, let alone cats. Everyone in authority—government officials, scientists, and food industry groups—appeared to be more concerned about the health of the meat and meat processing industries than about the health of the British public.

The United States government had its own problems with mad cow disease. In its November report, the Science Board noted that when BSE first appeared in Europe,

consumers and the industry looked to the FDA to ensure that
the disease would not spread to the US through the animal feed
that FDA regulates. But Agency officials were denied funds
that would bring the feed industry into compliance with new
regulations and the disease did appear in a few cows in the US.
Perhaps if the small sums requested by FDA had been provided, Japan and other countries would not have cut off imports
of US beef and American producers would not have suffered
multibillion dollar losses. To this day, the BSE research program . . . remains seriously underfunded.

This brings us back to the FDA's lack of resources, but also
raises another issue: the profound loss of confidence in the food
supply caused by the BSE events. Did the pet food crisis have a
similar effect? So it seems. In a poll conducted by the Food
Marketing Institute in January 2006—consider this as a base-
line—82% of respondents said they were completely confident
or somewhat confident in the safety of the food supply. One year
later, shortly after the outbreak of cases of *E. coli* O157:H7 in
bagged spinach, the percentage had dropped to 66%. On March
31, two weeks after Menu Foods' first recall announcement, the
figure fell to 60%.

By December 2007, only about half of respondents to a survey
conducted by a communications firm reported confidence in the
safety of the food supply. That survey asked respondents to rank
their sources of information about food choices by degree of trust.
The most trusted source? I could hardly believe the answer: food
activists. The largest percentage of respondents (66%) ranked
food activists as the most reliable sources of information, closely
followed by retail grocers (62%). Even food manufacturers (53%)
ranked higher than government, as only 47% of respondents said

they trusted the U.S. government's advice about food choices. As a bit of an activist myself, I particularly appreciate the first of these results—recognition at long last—but am dismayed by the declining trust in government. Surely a strong, independent, well-funded FDA would better protect the food supply; a better protected food supply would help restore public trust; and trust in the food supply would be good for business as well as for the health of people and pets.

And that brings me to the last repercussion: the effects of the recalls on the pet food industry, pet owners, and everything else that falls into the category of pet food politics.

20

....

REPERCUSSION #4:
PET FOOD POLITICS

Advocates for the safety of the human food supply consistently call for standard safety procedures to be applied to all foods, from farm to table. These, we say, should be administered by a single food safety agency that encompasses the present oversight functions of the FDA, USDA, and other federal agencies. Advocates for pets want nothing less for pet foods. The pet food recalls demonstrated why such proposals deserve serious consideration.

The commercial pet food industry, however, deeply distrusts and opposes the idea of further regulation. In April, the president of the Pet Food Institute, a trade association for the industry, made this point while blaming the FDA for the crisis:

> We do feel that if FDA had been able to specify earlier on what ingredient was under investigation that we could have assisted them in finding and removing affected products from commerce in a more timely fashion . . . pet food produced for the United States is among the most regulated products on store shelves today . . . this was not a problem we believe more regu-

lations can fix . . . The answer to this problem is not additional regulation, rather it is enhanced communication.

Many pet owners would disagree. They might appreciate better communication, but also want better regulation, particularly of the contents and labeling of pet foods. The recalls provided plenty of evidence to explain why pet owners want the labels of pet foods to disclose far more about the contents of the products than they currently do. Pet food labels in 2007 followed the rules for labels on animal feed products. Pet owners, however, were calling for the far more informative "nutrition facts" labels that appear on human food products. The differences in label formats reflect the different histories of the FDA's Center for Food Safety and Applied Nutrition, which oversees the human food supply, and its Center for Veterinary Medicine, which oversees farm feed and pet food.

In September, Congress responded. In the odd way in which our government often does such things, Congress attached food safety provisions to the Prescription Drug User Fee Act. (All one can say is, why not, if that's what works.) These provisions include two sections that deal with pet foods, one for regulation, "Ensuring the Safety of Pet Food," and one for communication, "Ensuring Efficient and Effective Communications during a Recall." On the regulation side, Congress said the FDA is to work with relevant stakeholder groups to establish ingredient, labeling, and processing standards for pet food. On the communication side, the FDA is to develop early warning systems for identifying outbreaks of illness in pets along the lines of those run by the Centers for Disease Control and Prevention.

The government of Canada also responded to the recalls by

initiating a review of its pet food responsibilities. The Canadian Food Inspection Agency (CFIA), which regulates imports, created a hold-and-test program for Chinese shipments entering Canada. In October 2007, the Canadian government established a website to allow the public to search for recalled food products and, in December, announced a new food and consumer safety action plan that would mandate product recalls, fines, and better safeguards. By early 2008, however, nothing much had happened with the plan. As explained by a spokesperson for the agency, Canada doesn't regulate pet food: "We're the Canadian Food Inspection Agency. We deal with food—and food is for humans."

As for the United States, it was too soon in early 2008 to know whether the new initiatives would translate into meaningful improvements, but its actions did give reason for hope that the recalls might lead to long-lasting benefits.

Besides increasing the pressure to improve standards, labels, and communication, the recalls had other effects on the pet food industry. Of these, four merit special consideration: the economic impact, the legal challenges, the movement toward alternative feeding methods, and the emergence of bloggers as a major influence on public understanding of pet food issues.

The Economic Impact

In the immediate aftermath of the recall, sales of pet foods dropped by more than 30%. Faced with the need for damage control, the Pet Food Institute (PFI) hired a public relations firm to manage its communications strategy. The institute placed full-page newspaper advertisements addressed to "Dear Pet Lovers." These said, "Our hearts go out to those affected and we vow to work tirelessly to continue our efforts to keep your pets safe and healthy." In a further effort to restore trust in the safety of the products, PFI announced the formation of the National Pet Food Commission to investigate the recall and to recommend steps to be taken to "build on safety and quality standards already in place for pet food."

Seeing the crisis as a wake-up call, pet food companies improved oversight, did their own ingredient testing, checked the accuracy of their product labels, and began tracking where their ingredients came from—all changes for the better. Such changes, should they last, also can be counted as positive results of these events. Companies also worked on public relations. They took care to distance themselves from Menu Foods and announced that they would only be buying ingredients made in America.

In November, the National Pet Food Commission submitted its report to the PFI. The report contained two sets of recommendations, some for the institute itself and some for the pet food industry. The commission's suggestions for the PFI were expressed in gentle terms such as "develop," "use," "explore," "approach," "volunteer," and, occasionally, "establish oversight." Some examples: "Develop a model emergency response plan . . . Volunteer to host a vulnerability assessment exercise . . . Explore mechanisms to communicate identities of recalled products to consumers." The commission's recommendations to manufacturers encouraged cooperation, communication, and updating of methods, as can be seen in these examples: "Reevaluate current sampling and testing protocols . . . and establish ongoing communication links with colleges of veterinary medicine."

If these suggestions do not seem to address more fundamental problems or the pet food industry's need to get its act together, improve its practices, and lobby for stronger and more trustworthy regulations, it is surely because PFI represents pet food companies, not pet owners. The commission's purpose was not to stir up the industry. The commission's principal—perhaps only—purpose was public relations. This became clear in December when *Newsweek* interviewed Gene Grabowski, vice president of Levick Strategic Communications, "who worked damage control on the national pet-food recalls." Grabowski explained the three rules of public relations: (1) take responsibility and (2) control the pictures. Here is his (3):

> Create some kind of structure, some kind of system to study the situation and act responsibly to implement it. I handled the pet-food crisis. One of the things we did at the pet-food association was to create a national pet-food commission that issued a report at [the] end of three months. By creating a commission we acted quickly and responsibly. We had full-page ads and presented it [the report] to Congress. It's not enough in today's world to just do the right thing, but to also show the world that you are doing the right thing.

If the impetus for the commission's report was to restore consumer trust in pet food products, it was going to take more than public relations to do it. PFI had its work cut out for it. The most evident sign of loss of trust was a continuing decline in sales. Hardest hit were Iams products, made by P&G. These experienced a 17% loss in sales in the first few months, a hit so serious that investment analysts advised P&G to divest itself of its pet food lines. Pet foods, as noted earlier, comprised just a small fraction of P&G's annual sales. Indeed, analysts said that any company distrusted by customers should be considered vulnerable to buyouts and takeovers.

On average, sales of private-label brands fell by 15%. In contrast, Hill's Science Diet, sold mainly through veterinarians, did better. Its sales held steady, perhaps because the company resorted to a lot more than public relations to handle the crisis. On March 30, after melamine had been identified in ChemNutra wheat gluten, Hill's immediately recalled Prescription Diet products made with that ingredient. Officials of the company told my colleague, Dr. Malden Nesheim, that within two hours of learning about the melamine contamination, the company contacted every client to which it shipped product and within a few days personally called every one of the 16,000 veterinarians who sell its products.

By the end of December 2007, Menu Foods' unit price had fallen to 10% of its value a year earlier (see Figure 2). In February 2008, the company announced a net loss of $62 million (Canadian) on $245 million in sales for the 2007 fiscal year; in comparison, the company had made a profit of $6.4 million on sales of $356 million a year earlier. Overall pet food sales had not yet returned to pre-recall levels, and retail companies like PetSmart expected the shortfall to be in the "tens of millions of dollars." These losses, severe as they might be, did not include the costs of litigation. At the Pet Expo in February 2008, I was told that Menu Foods had approached most large commercial pet food makers with an offer to sell but that none were willing to take on the risk of liability. The costs of defending against or settling lawsuits, to understate the matter, were likely to be substantial.

The Legal Challenges

Within days of the first recall announcements, pet owners in Canada and the United States filed lawsuits individually and as part of class actions. Menu Foods alone faced 50 lawsuits by the end of April and by October, the number exceeded 100. Under traditional laws in the United States, which treat pets as property, awards for damages would be limited to the amount owners paid for their pets and the subsequent costs of food and veterinary care. But trial lawyers and animal rights advocates had more ambitious ideas. They were hoping to use the suits to induce the courts to allow additional judgments for emotional damage. Such damages would encompass not only the grief experienced by owners (in this context, guardians) as a result of losing their pets, but also the distress caused by the pet food companies' apparent indifference to the suffering of their animals.

Some legal authorities believe that Canadian court decisions provide precedents for awarding compensation based on the extent of pain and suffering brought on by the illness or death of a pet. They see the traditional view of animals as property shifting to one that recognizes the role of pets in people's lives. And because companies use the emotional attachment of owners to pets to market their products, they ought to be liable for emotional damages. For companies subject to the lawsuits, the idea of compensation for emotional costs must be daunting. It could take pet liability damages into the stratospheric heights of compensation for human liability.

Lawyers also used the pet food recalls as an opportunity to file class-action suits on additional legal grounds. One suit, for example, accused pet food companies of engaging in misleading advertising. How? The labels of pet foods failed to warn buyers about the potential health risks of the products' ingredients. In February 2008, a U.S. judicial panel consolidated 120 class-action lawsuits filed in 20 states and assigned the consolidated case to the U.S.

District Judge in Camden, New Jersey. After weeks of mediation, the defendants—Menu Foods and dozens of pet food makers and sellers—were still arguing with the plaintiffs' lawyers about the terms of a possible settlement. But the judge said the parties had to reach agreement by April 1 or be ready to go to trial. On April 1, lawyers agreed in principle to settle but would not disclose the terms until they were approved by the U.S. and Canadian courts.

While lawyers at pet food companies were struggling to prepare defenses against litigation, other officials were using the lawsuits as an excuse to maintain secrecy about their companies' part in the recall, even when secrecy did not seem to be necessary. Here is one example: I was curious to know more about P&G's role in the recall because that company seemed so far ahead of everyone else in hearing about sick cats, recalling its products, forcing Menu Foods to issue a recall, and identifying melamine as the toxin. P&G, I thought, should be proud of these achievements. I wondered how the company had managed to accomplish them and why it wasn't letting its loyal Iams and Eukanuba customers in on the secret.

As it happened, I met a former CEO of the company at a dinner event who said he would see what he could do to get my questions answered. Indeed, I was soon contacted by Kurt Wiengand, P&G Pet Care's associate director for global external relations. In response to my admittedly picky queries (I was hoping he could confirm the dates on which events occurred), he sent me a collection of publicly available documents, all of which I had already seen, along with this message: "Unfortunately, P&G is involved in litigation concerning this issue, so I cannot comment on the details of the case at this time . . . Throughout this situation, our focus was on protecting pets and helping their owners. We appreciate your interest in telling this story and hope it provides some instructive lessons." Yes, I hope so too.

Indeed, some instructive lessons arrived in February 2008, when the FDA announced that its investigations had led a federal grand jury in Kansas City, Missouri, to indict the owners or managers of Xuzhou Anying, Suzhou Textiles, and ChemNutra "for their roles in a scheme to import products purported to be wheat gluten into the United States." The indictments accuse Xuzhou Anying's manager, Mao Lijun (called Mao Linzhun in the documents) of deliberately passing off wheat flour laced with melamine as wheat gluten, something he had apparently admitted to Chinese authorities in April.

Beyond that, the crucial charges dealt with the arcane matter of switching label codes on international shipments. It seems that an obscure (at least to me) group called the World Customs Organization develops "Harmonized Commodity Description and Coding Systems" that assign code numbers to thousands of items involved in international trade. These systems require shipments of wheat gluten to be labeled with code 1109. Under Chinese law, materials marked with that particular code must be inspected before they can be exported. In contrast, collagen and "other protein substances and their derivatives, not otherwise specified" are assigned code 3504; materials labeled with this code do not require inspection. The indictment accuses the owners of ChemNutra, Stephen Miller and his wife Sally Qing Miller, of conspiring with Suzhou Textiles to import wheat gluten deliberately labeled with code 3504 to evade Chinese inspectors.

As best I can determine from the indictment documents, which make interesting if not always illuminating reading, ChemNutra ran into problems with its usual supplier of wheat gluten in late September 2006. Beginning on November 8 of that year, and continuing until March 14, 2007, ChemNutra imported wheat gluten labeled with harmonized systems (HS) code 3504 from Suzhou Textiles. In the occasionally poetic language of the indictment:

> It was further a part of the conspiracy and scheme and artifice to defraud that the defendants hired a customs broker in Kansas City, Missouri, to assist them in importing the Chinese manufactured wheat gluten into the United States and, when HS code 3504.0090 appeared on Chinese documents . . . the defendants instructed the customs broker to use HS code 1109.0000 when completing the paperwork needed to import the Chinese wheat gluten into the United States.

I cannot tell from reading the indictments who knew what, when, or whether the Millers were guilty of fraud or were just trying to be expedient in meeting their customers' needs under difficult circumstances. The courts, no doubt, will sort out such matters in good time. What is abundantly clear from these documents, however, is the frustration experienced by importers of food ingredients from China and the difficulties involved in overseeing the quality of those ingredients—even when the importer is, like Mrs. Miller, of Chinese origin and fluent in the language and culture of the exporting country.

The Alternative Pet Food Movement

Before Blue Buffalo—a "natural" brand—was faced with the problem of its own recalls, the company benefited from a sales increase of 50%. Other makers of pet foods based on free-range meat, organic vegetables, and brown rice reported sales increases of as much as 90%. Commercial companies responded immediately by introducing 38 new pet foods labeled as containing no wheat.

Nevertheless, the recalls shook the foundations of the entire industry, one that many believed needed just such a jolt. Distrust of commercial pet foods induced owners to get foods tested on their own and to seek alternative ways to feed their pets. In answer to the question, "Can you recommend any safe pet food products?" readers of some Internet sites were told things like "No . . . it is impossible to endorse any commercial pet food product as being safe. The only recommendation we are able to make with a clear conscience is to make your own pet food at home." Pet owners had plenty of options for doing just that. Advocates for raw food diets placed advertisements saying, "Doesn't the latest news on pet-food recalls make you want to BARF? It should." BARF refers to the increasingly popular Biologically Appropriate Raw Food or Bones and Raw Food diets, which in this context were certain to be free of melamine. Recipe books for do-it-yourself pet foods flew off the shelves, as did pet food brands labeled "natural," "organic," "Kosher," or "holistic." At the Pet Expo in February 2008, the makers of raw and natural pet foods and treats smiled happily when I asked them how their businesses were doing. As *Nutrition Business Journal* explained, "What's bad for the mainstream pet food industry is proving a bonanza for makers of natural and organic dog and cat foods." The rationale for this bonanza is easy to explain, as shown in Figure 6.

The companies that derived the greatest benefit were those that not only behaved responsibly but also made efforts to let their customers know what they were doing. *Nutrition Business*

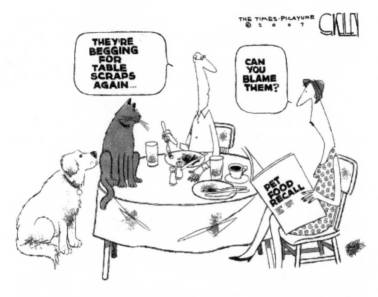

Figure 6. The origin of the Good Pet Food movement. The pet food recalls stimulated rejection of commercial foods and interest in home cooking for cats and dogs. The drawing appeared in the New Orleans *Times-Picayune,* March 23, 2007. *Steve Kelley Editorial Cartoon* ©2007 Steve Kelley.

Journal singled out Castor & Pollux Pet Works, maker of organic and natural pet foods, for particular praise. That company immediately tested its products and found them free of melamine but recalled them anyway. It also contacted all of its major accounts within a day and offered rebates to customers. Natural Balance developed tests for melamine and cyanuric acid and posted the results on its website, where customers could check specific products by clicking on a "buy with confidence" banner. With that system online, the company's sales, which had gone flat after the recall, recovered and rose to record levels.

Pet Food Express, a chain of retail stores in the San Francisco Bay Area, removed all products made by Menu Foods, whether or not the products had been recalled. The company required manufacturers to provide the results of melamine tests if they wanted their products reinstated. Most did, but the makers of Iams (P&G) and Science Diet (Hill's) refused, and Pet Food Express refused to stock their canned foods. The company's "calm, reasoned response to the recall" explains why it was named by *Pet Product News* as retailer of the year in 2007–2008. In January 2008, I spoke with one of the company's owners, Michael Levy, and chief operating officer Terry Lim about why they had decided to take these actions. They explained that their previous experience with the Petcurean recall in 2003 (see Chapter 2) convinced them that pet food cannot be considered safe until it is proven to be. As Terry Lim put it, their customers want more than quality assurance. They also want emotional assurance. And doing the right thing is good for business.

Such sentiments are expressed even more forcefully by Nancy Kerns, editor of *The Whole Dog Journal,* which rates dog foods on several criteria, origin of manufacture among them. For her readers, the critical issue is *transparency.*

> That's what the pet food recalls of early 2007 taught us to value in a pet food company . . . Some companies "got it," and responded immediately with up-to-the-minute updates . . . In our view, the best ones were the companies that stated immediately where their foods were made, where their ingredients came from, and what they were doing to ensure their products were safe. But many other companies stone-walled, insisting that their products were safe but refusing to offer any corroborating evidence!

The American College of Veterinary Nutrition, a professional organization of veterinarians trained in nutrition, reflected the dismay of the commercial pet food industry over the critique of the industry expressed in comments like these, and over consumers' search for alternative foods, in a statement on April 5, 2007:

> This incident has affected us deeply . . . However, the seemingly ever-changing news about the pet food recall has . . . allowed for wild speculation about the safety and wholesomeness of commercial pet foods in general and mistrust of both the industry and government oversight of the industry. Some parties have taken advantage of this dire situation to enflame these concerns so they may advance their own cause or agendas . . . [We] advise those pet owners considering home formulation of diets for their pets to be duly cautious. Many recipes found on the web or elsewhere, even from well-meaning sources, may not be complete and balanced, creating the possibility of significant long-term harm to animals fed diets based on these recipes.

Pet owners might consider the threat of melamine to be anything but "wild speculation" and the behavior of the companies and government to provide ample grounds for mistrust and the need for safer alternatives. It is certainly true that commercial pet foods provide complete and balanced nutrition (they have to), and, as the college points out, "It simply is not in the best interest of companies to want to sell potentially unsafe product." But I suspect that the college's opinion that "as a whole, the pet food industry has been duly diligent and has acted responsibly in its response to the incident" is open to debate. Among their other consequences, the recalls encouraged scrutiny of the source and quality of ingredients in pet foods, matters that pet food companies would just as soon keep to themselves.

In revising *Food Politics* for its new edition in 2007, I wrote about food advocacy as a new social movement. This movement, I explained, may be fragmented, uncoordinated, and spontaneous, but it exhibits all of the hallmarks of democracy at its best—of the people, by the people, and for the people. The overall food movement incorporates a wide range of smaller movements, all of them devoted to creating meaningful alternatives to the current industrialized and globalized food system. Consider, for example, the Farm Aid movement (which supports food that is good for health, clean for the environment, and fair to its producers), the Slow Food movement (the opposite of fast food), the organic foods movement, the locavore movement, and the animal welfare movement. These separate movements aim to promote the physical, moral, and ethical health of humans, food animals, and the environment. To this collection of mini-movements, we can now add the Good Pet Food movement, with its goals of health, sound ethics, environmental sustainability—and, now more than ever, advocacy. May it flourish.

The New Influence of Bloggers

If the Menu Foods recalls made pet owners desperate for alternatives, bloggers deserve much credit for fueling the Good Pet Food movement. For pet owners, the most horrendous problem with the recall was the absence of information about which products were safe. Into the breach stepped bloggers. Volunteers on sites such as PetConnection.com and Itchmo.com produced daily lists of recalled and unrecalled foods, tracked pet illnesses and deaths, and provided immediate links to company press releases, pet food industry websites, veterinary information, and FDA and other government website postings of recall notices, tele-conferences, hearings, and news releases. I spent several days reading through the archives of blog sites and was impressed by the quality of the information. The sites are a treasure trove of data, documents, and otherwise unavailable resources, and it is no wonder that they were so widely used by pet owners as well as reporters, government officials, pet food company officials, and lawyers. Among the documents sent to me by the P&G official, for example, were blog postings from PetConnection.com, an indication that P&G must have been tracking the site.

The pet recall sites dealt with personal as well as political matters, and at least one was entirely devoted to the victims of the contaminated foods. That site invited pet owners to create memorials to animals that died as a result of eating the tainted food. By the end of 2007, more than 900 owners had posted photographs and memorials to their deceased pets (another self-reported estimate of the body count). Overall, the sites were so useful that media experts judged the pet bloggers as having changed the practice of journalism, and much for the better, making it more immediate, less competitive, and more focused on the search for truth.

In Chapter 16, I mentioned how the FDA recognized this change by reaching out to bloggers. I learned about this effort early in November 2007, when I received an e-mail invitation from the FDA's website management staff to participate in a November 14 teleconference to discuss the newly announced Food Protection Plan. The invitation said, "As commentators on food, health, and related topics, we know you are in touch with public concerns about food safety and we are interested in hearing from you. So for the first time, the FDA is organizing a teleconference specifically for bloggers. I hope you will join us." I was pleased to do so.

FDA Commissioner Andrew von Eschenbach began the teleconference by explaining its purpose. The FDA, he said, wants to communicate with the people it serves. It would continue to use traditional channels but also wanted to take advantage of emerging venues such as the Internet. The FDA, he told us, realizes that bloggers have seized this opportunity for communication and dialogue, so "we wanted to reach out to you. Just as I have brown bag sessions with media . . . we wanted to offer bloggers a similar kind of dialogue." In this sense, the FDA was according bloggers the same status as reporters on national newspapers or magazines.

I think the FDA was smart to do this. Here is one reason. On April 3, less than three weeks after the first announcement of the recall and long before its full implications could even have been imagined, Christie Keith, who writes a syndicated pet advocacy column for Pet Connection and is a regular columnist for the *San Francisco Chronicle,* took on critics—and there were many at the time—who thought pet owners, the FDA, and the media were making far too much fuss over a few cats and dogs. Ms. Keith quoted one such critic, Rosie O'Donnell, then cohost of the daytime talk show *The View:*

> Fifteen cats and one dog have died, and it's been all over the news. And you know, since that date, 29 soldiers have died, and we haven't heard much about them. No. I think that we have the wrong focus in the country. That when pets are killed in America from some horrific poisoning accident, 16 of them, it's all over the news and people are like, "The kitty! It's so sad." Twenty-nine sons and daughters killed since that day, it's not newsworthy. I don't understand.

Here is Christie Keith's prescient response:

> In fact, Rosie didn't understand. She didn't understand that the
> same government she blames for sending America's sons and
> daughters to die in Iraq is the government that told her only 15
> animals had died, and that the story was about a pet "poisoning
> accident" and not a systemic failure of FEMA-esque propor-
> tions . . . It may turn out that our dogs and cats were the canar-
> ies in the coal mine of an enormous system failure—one that
> could have profound impacts on American food manufacturing
> and safety in the years to come.

In this case, I prefer to think that the warning comes from a
Chihuahua, not a canary, but the message is the same. If we want
our global food system to provide safe food for everyone, ensuring the safety of pets is as good a place as any to start. Protection
of the health and safety of society's most vulnerable members is
the cornerstone of American democracy. In this particular incident, the most vulnerable were cats and dogs. We would do well
to heed their warning.

APPENDIX

....

THE MELAMINE RECALLS LIST

The FDA's final list of brands of recalled cat and dog foods appears as an Excel spreadsheet of 1,171 lines. The list is difficult to use, not only because it is hard to read but also because it includes products recalled because of *Salmonella* as well as melamine contamination. Table 8 is derived from the FDA's list. It lists nearly 200 brands of cat foods and dog foods recalled because their labels listed wheat gluten (no asterisk) or rice protein concentrate (indicated with an asterisk), although the products actually contained wheat flour contaminated with melamine and by-products such as cyanuric acid. These contaminants form crystals that block kidney function.

The FDA's complete recall list is much more extensive than indicated here. It provides the names of individual product lines within each brand. Table 9 provides one example—the list of Iams cat food products recalled by Procter & Gamble. The number of items on this list is in no way atypical. For example, the recalled products included 14 varieties of Science Diet cat foods, 20 of Nutro Natural Choice cat foods, 27 of Alpo dog foods, and

28 of Ol' Roy Canada dog foods. Iams also recalled 23 types of dog foods. Altogether, the FDA estimated that 5,300 separate products were involved in the melamine recalls.

The FDA site and that of the American Veterinary Medical Association provide links to company websites, recall notices, and information about specific products.

Table 8. Cat and dog food brands recalled for melamine contamination, March 16 – May 23, 2007

Cat Foods	Dog Foods
Americas Choice, Preferred Pet	ALPO
Authority	Americas Choice, Preferred Pet
Best Choice	Authority
Blue Buffalo Co*	Award
Cats Choice	Best Choice
Co-Op Gold	Big Bet
Companion	Big Red
Compliments	Bloom
Demolulas Market Basket	Blue Buffalo*
Demolulas Market Basket†	Bruiser
Despar	Cadillac
Diamond Pet Foods*	Canine Caviar Pet Foods*
Doctors Foster & Smith	Champion Breed Lg Biscuit
Doctors Foster & Smith*	Champion Breed Peanut Butter Biscuits
Eukanuba Cat Cuts and Flaked	Co-Op Gold
Eukanuba Morsels in Gravy	Companion
Evolve	Companion's Best Multi-Flavor Biscuit
Evolve†	Compliments
Fame	Costco/Kirkland Signature*
Feline Classic	Demoulas Market Basket
Feline Cuisine	Diamond Pet Foods

Table 8 *(continued)*

Cat Foods	Dog Foods
Fine Feline Cat	Diamond Pet Foods*
Food Lion	Doctors Foster & Smith
Foodtown	Doctors Foster & Smith*
Giant Companion	Dollar General
Giant Eagle	Eukanuba Can Dog Chunks in Gravy
Hannaford	Eukanuba Pouch Dog Bites in Gravy
Harmony Farms*	Food Lion
Health Diet Cat Food	Giant Companion
Hill Country Fare	Gravy Train
Hill's Prescription Diet	Grreat Choice
Hy-Vee	Hannaford
Hy-Vee†	Happy Tails
Iams Cat Slices and Flakes	Harmony Farms*
Iams Select Bites	Harmony Farms Treats*
J.E. Mondou	Health Diet Gourmet Cuisine
La Griffe	Hill Country Fare
Laura Lynn	Hy-Vee
Li'l Red	Hy-Vee†
Lick Your Chops	Iams Can Chunky Formula
Lick Your Chops*	Iams Can Small Bites Formula
Loving Meals	Iams Dog Select Bites
Master Choice	Jerky Treats Beef Flavored Dog Snacks
Medi-Cal	La Griffe
Meijer's Main Choice	Laura Lynn
Natural Balance*	Loving Meals
Natural Ultramix	Master Choice
Nu Pet	Meijer's Main Choice
Nutriplan	Mighty Dog
Nutro	Mixables
Nutro Max Cat Gourmet Classics	Mulligan Stew Pet Food*
Nutro Max Gourmet Classics	Natural Balance*
Nutro Natural Choice	Natural Life

(continued)

Table 8 *(continued)*

Cat Foods	Dog Foods
Nutro Products	Natural Way
Paws	Nu Pet
Performatrin Ultra	Nutriplan
Pet Pride	Nutro
Pet Pride/Good n Meaty	Nutro Ultra
Pounce	Nutro Max
Presidents Choice	Nutro Natural Choice
Price Chopper	Nurture
Priority Canada	Ol' Roy
Priority US	Ol' Roy 4-Flavor Lg Biscuits
Publix	Ol' Roy Canada
Roche Brothers	Ol' Roy Peanut Butter Biscuits
Roundy's	Ol' Roy Puppy
Royal Canin*	Ol' Roy US
Royal Canin Veterinary Diet*	Paws
Save-A-Lot Special Blend	Perfect Pals Large Biscuits
Schnucks	Performatrin Ultra
Science Diet Feline Cuts Adult	Pet Essentials
Science Diet Feline Cuts Kitten	Pet Life
Science Diet Feline Cuts Mature Adult 7+	Pet Pride/Good n Meaty
Science Diet Feline Savory Cuts Can	Presidents Choice
Sophistacat	Price Chopper
Special Kitty Canada	Priority Canada
Special Kitty US	Priority US
Springfield Prize	Publix
Sprout	Roche Brothers
Stop & Shop Companion	Royal Canin*
Stuzzy Gold	Royal Canin Veterinary Diet*
Triumph	Save-A-Lot Choice Morsels
Wegmans	Schnuck's
Weis Total Pet	Schnucks†
Western Family Canada	Shep

Table 8 *(continued)*

Cat Foods	Dog Foods
Western Family US	Shep Dog
White Rose	Shop Rite
Winn Dixie	SmartPak*
Your Pet	Springfield Prize
	Sprout
	Stater Brothers
	Stater Brothers Large Biscuits
	Stop & Shop Companion
	Tops Companion
	Triumph
	Truly
	Weis Total Pet
	Western Family Canada
	Western Family US
	White Rose
	Winn Dixie
	Your Pet

Source: FDA. Search for pet food recalls. Updated January 22, 2008, at www.accessdata .fda.gov/scripts/petfoodrecall/#All.

*Indicates products recalled because their ingredients included rice protein concentrate; all others were products made according to formulas that included wheat gluten.

†Indicates a different set of recalled products from the same brand.

Table 9. Iams cat foods recalled by Procter & Gamble, March 16, 2007

Slices and Flakes in Cans

    Slices: turkey in gravy, 3 and 6 oz. (adult)

    Slices: beef in gravy, 3 and 6 oz. (adult)

    Slices: chicken in gravy, 3 and 6 oz. (adult)

    Slices: turkey in gravy, 3 oz. (kitten)

    Flakes: tuna and ocean white fish in sauce, 3 and 6 oz. (adult)

    Flakes: salmon in sauce, 3 and 6 oz. (adult)

    Variety pack slices: chicken and beef in gravy (adult)

    Variety pack flakes: tuna and ocean white fish and salmon in sauce (adult)

Select Bites in Pouches (3 oz.)

    Beef in gravy (adult)

    Chicken and wild rice in gravy (adult)

    Chicken in gravy (adult)

    Turkey in gravy (adult)

    Salmon in sauce (adult)

    Tuna in sauce (adult)

    Chicken in gravy (kitten)

    Tuna in sauce (weight control)

    Chicken in gravy (active maturity)

    Variety pack with beef, chicken, and turkey

    Variety pack with salmon and tuna

    Variety pack with chicken and turkey

Source: FDA. Search for pet food recalls. Updated January 22, 2008, at www
.accessdata.fda.gov/scripts/petfoodrecall/#All.

NOTES

All Internet addresses were accessible in April 2008 unless otherwise stated.

Introduction

p. 8 *This account is mostly* Pet food recall claims No. 1 "spot" in annual survey of America's food editors. PR Newswire, December 17, 2007, at http://sev.pr newswire.com/food-beverages/20071217/NYM00717122007-1.html.

1. A Recall to Break All Records

p. 9 *On or about February 20* The date is in dispute. The FDA's March 19 teleconference gave the date as February 20 (www.fda.gov/oc/opacom/hot topics/petfood/transcript031907.pdf), whereas Menu's CEO Paul Henderson used February 22 at congressional hearings on April 24 (transcript of Paul Henderson's testimony to the Subcommittee on Oversight and Investigations, House Committee on Energy and Commerce, April 24, 2007, at http://energy commerce.house.gov/cmte_mtgs/110-oi-hrg.042407.food.supply.shtml).

p. 9 *While these calls* Pet Food Industry (September 2007) lists laboratories that perform nutrient analyses and microbiological assays; that test for antibiotics, pesticides, genetic modifications, and antioxidants; and that evaluate claims for "complete and balanced," palatability, digestibility, and bioavailability. Some give locations and websites, but others do not.

p. 10 *Later, in explaining* Transcript of Paul Henderson's testimony to the Subcommittee on Oversight and Investigations, House Committee on Energy and Commerce, April 24, 2007, at http://energycommerce.house.gov/cmte _mtgs/110-oi-hrg.042407.food.supply.shtml.

p. 11 *About wheat gluten* The two principal proteins in wheat gluten are gliadin and glutenin. Tsai M. Un-American pet food: why do we put Chinese wheat gluten in fido's kibble? *Slate,* April 2, 2007, at www.slate.com/id/2163235.

p. 11 *The next day, March 9* Statement of Donald Smith, dean of the College of Veterinary Medicine, Cornell University. Transcript of FDA press conference on the pet food recall, March 30, 2007, at www.fda.gov/oc/opacom/ hottopics/petfood/transcript033007.pdf.

p. 12 *On March 13* Procter & Gamble. Veterinary Quality Assurance Task Force report, March 29, 2007, at http://us.iams.com/iams/global/Vet_Quality _Assurance_Report.htm. P&G scientists corroborated other details in off-the-record conversations.

p. 12 *The next afternoon* Menu Foods Income Fund announces precautionary dog and cat food recall (press release), March 16, 2007, at www.menufoods .com.

p. 13 *Although this was* Within a year, the pet food recall was upstaged by a recall of 143 million pounds of ground beef. See Martin A. Largest recall of ground beef is ordered. *New York Times,* February 18, 2008, at www.nytimes .com/2008/02/18/business/18recall.html?_r=1&st=cse&sq=meat+recall&scp=1 &oref=slogin.

2. A Brief Historical Digression

p. 15 *Note my choice* FDA. Background and definitions at www.fda.gov/oc/ po/firmrecalls/recall_defin.html. FDA, Center for Veterinary Medicine. Types of regulatory actions, September 18, 1998, at www.fda.gov/cvm/Policy _Procedures/3601.pdf.

p. 19 *Petcurean Pet Nutrition* The Petcurean website is www.petcurean.com. The October 22, 2003, recall was reclassified as a market withdrawal on April 4, 2004; it is posted on the FDA recall site at www.fda.gov/oc/po/firmrecalls/pet curean10_03.html. See Smith AJ, Stenske KA, Bartges JW, et al. Diet-associated hepatic failure and immune-mediated hemolytic anemia in a Weimaraner. *Journal of Veterinary Emergency and Critical Care* 2006;16(S1):S42–S47.

p. 19 *But the FDA did* FDA. Memorandum: Go Natural dog and cat food recall, April 2, 2004, at http://69.20.19.211/cvm/Documents/HHEGoNatural.pdf.

p. 20 *Pet owners filed* See Rosynsky PT. Pet Food Express suing supplier over dog deaths. *Oakland Tribune,* April 6, 2007. Also, *Match vs. Pet Food*

Express, case # RG03–127285, Superior Court of the State of California in and for the County of Alameda, November 2, 2007, at http://apps.alameda.courts .ca.gov/fortecgi/fortecgi.exe?Servicename=DomainWebService&PageName= Image&ID=1&Parent=13103254&Action=19737599.

p. 20 *Even when the cause* York M. After recall of food, veterinarians at Cornell University rush to save poisoned dogs. *New York Times,* January 9, 2006. Kinnard M. Maker of tainted dog food settles. *Wall Street Journal,* January 5, 2008.

p. 22 *These pieces of evidence* Centers for Disease Control and Prevention. *Salmonella* Schwarzengrund outbreak investigation, August 2007, August 28, 2007, at www.cdc.gov/salmonella/schwarzengrund.html. FDA. Mars Petcare pet food recall: questions and answers, August 25, 2007, at www.fda.gov/bbs/ topics/NEWS/2007/NEW01689.html.

p. 23 *The Wal-Mart incident* Carney M. Wal-Mart: tests show dog treats tainted with melamine, *USA Today,* August 22, 2007, at http://blogs.usa today.com/ondeadline/2007/08/wal-mart-tests-.html. Wal-Mart. Statement on chicken jerky strips, August 22, 2007, at www.walmartfacts.com/articles/5241 .aspx. McCormick LW. FDA testing dog treats pulled from Wal-Mart shelves, August 23, 2007, at www.consumeraffairs.com/news04/2007/08/pet_food_recalls 68.html.

p. 23 *Nevertheless, the melamine* American Veterinary Medical Association. Media alert, September 14, 2007, at www.avma.org/press/media_alerts/070914 _jerky_treats.asp. Also, Lade DC. Bones? Yummies? Treats? Only in moderation, pet experts say. *South Florida Sun-Sentinal,* November 20, 2007.

p. 25 *Considering the millions* Wild Kitty Cat Food responds to FDA recall, February 21, 2007, at www.sys-con.com/read/339987_p.htm.

p. 25 *But it is not difficult* The ineffectiveness of recalls is best illustrated with meat. Recovery rates for 73 meat recalls in 2006 and 2007 averaged 44% but only 20% for five recalls involving illnesses among consumers. See Schmit J, Hansen B. Most recalled meat is never recovered, likely is eaten. *USA Today,* December 2, 2007.

p. 26 *In April, one month* FDA. FDA warns consumers that retailers may still have recalled pet food on shelves, April 12, 2007, at www.fda.gov/bbs/ topics/NEWS/2007/NEW01605.html. Nestle M, Nesheim MC. Additional information on melamine in pet food (letter). *Journal of the American Veterinary Medical Association* 2007;231:1647. Dr. Maslin's e-mail messages arrived on December 7, 2007.

3. The Sequence of Events

p. 28 *That may sound* See Christie Keith's unofficial transcript of testimony to the Subcommittee on Oversight and Investigations, House Committee on Energy and Commerce, April 24, 2007: "Diminished Capacity: Can the FDA Assure the Safety and Security of the Nation's Food Supply?" at www .petconnection.com/blog/2007/04/page/6. The transcript here is based on my review of the hearing video; the relevant dialogue begins at hour 3:44. No official transcript is available on the hearing site at http://energycommerce .house.gov/cmte_mtgs/110-oi-hrg.042407.food.supply.shtml.

p. 29 *Menu announced* P&G Pet Care announces voluntary participation in Menu Foods' nationwide U.S. and Canadian recall of specific canned and small foil pouch "wet" cat and dog foods (press release), March 16, 2007, at www.fda .gov/oc/po/firmrecalls/pg03_07.html.

4. What Is Menu Foods?

p. 42 *The pet food industry* Nesheim MC, Nestle M. Pet food. In: Allen G, Albala K, eds. *The Business of Food: Encyclopedia of the Food and Drink Industries.* Westport, CT: Greenwood Press, 2007:297–301. Top US pet food makers, 2006. In: Lazich RS, ed. *Market Share Reporter,* 2008, vol. 1:114. American Pet Products Manufacturing Association. Industry statistics and trends, at www .appma.org/press_industrytrends.asp. Johnson B. 100 leading national advertisers. *Advertising Age,* June 25, 2007.

p. 43 *Commercial pet foods* The Association of American Feed Control Officials (AAFCO) is an organization of state officials who regulate animal feed and pet foods in collaboration with the FDA. See www.aafco.org. Committees of the National Research Council have produced reports on dog nutrition since 1953 and on cat nutrition since 1978. The most recent is *Nutrient Requirements of Dogs and Cats* (Washington, DC: National Academies Press, 2006).

p. 45 *To make the different* Byron E. 101 Brand names, 1 manufacturer. *Wall Street Journal,* May 9, 2007.

p. 46 *Menu Foods was founded* Gillis C, Kingston A. How one supplier caused a huge crisis, and why it's just the tip of the iceberg. *Macleans,* April 30, 2007, at www.macleans.ca/business/companies/article.jsp?content=20070430 _104326_104326. Also see Austen I. Despite recall, pet food maker is still a large supplier. *New York Times,* March 22, 2007.

p. 48 *A few days after* Kwan J. Menu Foods again widens pet food recall. Reuters, April 10, 2007, at www.alertnet.org/thenews/newsdesk/N10443845 .htm.

p. 48 *Through much of* Schmit J. Pet-food industry feels side effects of recall. *USA Today,* July 11, 2007. Campbell C. After last spring's pet food scandal, Canada's Menu Foods fights for its life. *Macleans,* September 3, 2007, at www .macleans.ca/article.jsp?content=20070903_109055_109055&source=srch. Menu Foods cuts jobs, raises tainted-pet-food recall costs by $10M. *The Canadian Press,* October 11, 2007.

5. Menu's Muddled Response

p. 50 *The original recall* Menu Foods Income Fund. Press releases, March 16, 2007 to May 22, 2007, at www.menufoods.com/recall/index.html. Osborne WD. Recent pet food recall extremely complex. *FDA Veterinarian Newsletter,* 2007;22 (July 3): 1–4, at www.fda.gov/cvm/Documents/FDAVet2007VolXXII No2.pdf. Also see FDA. Import alert #99–29, detention without physical examination of all vegetable protein products from China for animal or human food use due to the presence of melamine and/or melamine analogs, July 31, 2007, at www.fda.gov/ora/fiars/ora_import_ia9929.html.

p. 51 *None of this helped* Staats J. Marin case confirms new tainted pet food. *Marin Independent Journal,* April 9, 2007. Mars, Incorporated to acquire Nutro Products, Inc. (press release), May 1, 2007, at www.nutroproducts.com/press 5-1-07mars.shtml.

p. 52 *Effective crisis management* Rosenblatt D. Handling customer complaints. In: Kvamme JL, Phillips TD, eds. *Petfood Technology.* Mt. Morris, IL: Watt Publishing, 2003:508–511. Sellers R. Recall realities: essential factors to think about in preparing for and handling a recall. *Petfood Industry,* October 2007:18–20.

p. 52 *In the event* Tan E. What you say: 93%. *Advertising Age,* April 2, 2007.

p. 53 *The March 16 recall* Zezima K. Pets' owners angered by delays in response. *New York Times,* March 22, 2007. Also see Henderson P. Transcript of testimony to the Subcommittee on Oversight and Investigations, House Committee on Energy and Commerce, April 24, 2007, at http://energycommerce .house.gov/cmte_mtgs/110-oi-hrg.042407.food.supply.shtml.

6. The Cat and Dog Body Count

p. 55 *The veterinary care system* Dahlberg CP. Rat poison in pet food. *Sacramento Bee,* March 24, 2007, at www.sacbee.com/267/story/143324.html. According to this account, from February 27 to March 2, the testing company gave 20 cats a choice of two foods, including a product not yet on the market, "to see how well they liked each one." The first cat died March 2 and the second on

March 5. Five cats died a few days later. The second test, on another 20 cats fed only the unmarketed food for two days, resulted in two deaths and one survivor with kidney damage. In a later test, most of 10 dogs refused food after the first day. This account is consistent with Henderson's congressional testimony. See Henderson P. Transcript of testimony to the Subcommittee on Oversight and Investigations, House Committee on Energy and Commerce, April 24, 2007, at http://energycommerce.house.gov/cmte_mtgs/110-oi-hrg.042407.food .supply.shtml.

p. 56 *Menu did not publicly* Burton TM. Amid pet-food recall, problem remains mystery. *Wall Street Journal,* March 19, 2007.

p. 58 *On March 26* Nation's largest pet insurer examines effects of pet food recall. PR Newswire, October 16, 2007, at http://sev.prnewswire.com/ health-care-hospitals/20071016/LATU05316102007-1.html. Also, Pet Connection, April 9, 2007, at www.petconnection.com/blog/2007/04/09/pet-food -recall-vin-follows-up-affirms-thousands-of-pets-potentially-affected. The Veterinary Information Network is at www.vin.com.

p. 59 *So if the numbers of* American Veterinary Medical Association. Researchers examine contaminants in food, deaths of pets. *javmaNews,* December 1, 2007, at www.avma.org/onlnews/javma/dec07/071201c-pf.asp.

7. A Toxic False Alarm: Aminopterin

p. 61 *After hearing about* Ramanujan K. Vet researchers seek to confirm presence of toxins in recalled pet food. *Cornell Chronicle,* March 29, 2007. New York State Department of Agriculture and Markets. Division of Food Laboratory, undated page at www.agmkt.state.ny.us/FL/FLHome.html. Gallagher J. Lab chief troubled by conflicting pet-food results. *Ithaca Journal,* April 3, 2007.

p. 62 *Pest control experts* Zezima K. Rat poison found in food linked to 14 animal deaths. *New York Times,* March 24, 2007.

8. At Last the Culprit: Melamine

p. 63 *By this time* FDA. Consumer update: FDA's ongoing pet food investigation, April 16, 2007, at www.fda.gov/consumer/updates/petfoodrecallup.html.

p. 63 *P&G scientists* Information about P&G scientific studies was discussed at a Procter & Gamble pet care conference, Cincinnati, OH, May 31, 2007, and corroborated independently by another P&G scientist. Identifying melamine was especially difficult because it was bound to cyanuric acid in the wheat gluten. Acid extraction broke up the melamine-cyanuric acid complexes (see Figure 3), releasing the two components in high enough concentration to be identified.

p. 64 *On Monday, March 26* Weise E, Schmit J. Pet deaths not easy to solve. *USA Today,* April 5, 2007. O'Flanigan R. Clues found in pet food deaths. *Guelph Mercury,* April 28, 2007. FDA's ongoing pet food investigation. *FDA Consumer Health Information,* April 16, 2007, at www.fda.gov/consumer/ updates/petfoodrecallup.html. Advion runs analyses using a chip-based integrated liquid chromatography/mass spectrometry system. See Advion's Tri-Versa NanoMate system essential in melamine analysis (press release), March 31, 2007, at www.advion.com/news-events/corporate/news/070331-triversa.php. Maxie G. Dealing with suspected pet food toxicities. *AHL* [Animal Health Laboratory] *LabNote* #13, March 27, 2007, at www.uoguelph.ca/labserv/units/ ahl/news_notes.cfm.

p. 65 *At teleconferences* See FDA press conference transcripts at www.fda .gov/oc/opacom/hottopics/petfood.html. Also see Goodman B. Pet food contained chemical found in plastic, F.D.A. says. *New York Times,* March 31, 2007. Bridges A. Cats fare worse in food contamination. Boston.com, March 30, 2007, at www.boston.com/business/articles/2007/03/31/cats_fare_worse_in_food _contamination. In December 2007, the FDA announced that Dr. Sundlof would switch jobs and leave his position at CVM to head the unit that regulates human food, the Center for Food Safety and Applied Nutrition.

p. 65 *So was the toxin* New York State Department of Agriculture and Markets. Statement from NYS Ag Commissioner Patrick Hooker, March 30, 2007, at www.agmkt.state.ny.us/ad/release.asp?releaseID=1599.

p. 66 *Regardless, melamine* Kegley S, Hill B, Orme S. PAN pesticide database. Pesticide Action Network, North America, 2000–2007, at www.pesticide info.org/List_NTPStudies.jsp?Rec_ID=PC35459. The odd appearance of the crystals and their effects on cats' kidneys were discussed during the March 30 FDA teleconference, at www.fda.gov/oc/opacom/hottopics/petfood.html.

p. 66 *At this point, the obvious* Roebuck K. Chinese criticized in pet food probe. *Pittsburgh Tribune-Review,* April 11, 2007, at http://pittsburghlive .com/x/pittsburghtrib/news/rss/s_502101.html. The USDA explains the provisions of the Animal Welfare Act and its various amendments at www.nal.usda .gov/awic/legislat/usdaleg1.htm#L5. Puschner B, Poppenga RH, Lowenstine LJ, et al. Assessment of melamine and cyanuric acid toxicity in cats. *Journal of Veterinary and Diagnostic Investigation* 2007;19:616–624.

9. Melamine: A Source of Nitrogen

p. 70 *Melamine and cyanuric*   See AOAC International. *Official Methods of Analysis of AOAC International,* 18th ed., Arlington, VA: AOAC International, 2005.

p. 71 *Melamine is cheap*   For a quick introduction to the Kjeldahl method, see http://en.wikipedia.org/wiki/Kjeldahl_method. An apparent protein content of 75% requires the addition of melamine at a concentration of roughly 18% (18 grams/100 grams). Wheat flour is 10 grams protein/100 grams, so another 65 grams of protein is needed. Melamine is 66.6% nitrogen, so 18 grams of melamine contain about 12 grams of nitrogen. Multiply 12 grams by 5.7, the conversion factor for wheat protein, to yield a bit more than 65 grams of apparent protein. Was anyone checking? Doubtful.

p. 71 *Wheat gluten may*   Radomski JL, Woodard G, Lehman AJ. The toxicity of flours treated with various "improving" agents. *Journal of Nutrition* 1948;36:15–25. Mellanby E. Further observations on the production of canine hysteria by flour treated with nitrogen trichloride (agene process). *British Medical Journal* 1947;2(4520):288–289.

p. 72 *As noted by the FDA*   Lipschitz WL, Stokey E. The mode of action of three new diuretics: melamine, adenine and formoguanamine. *Journal of Pharmacology and Experimental Therapeutics* 1945;83:235–249.

p. 73 *Beginning in the early*   Altona RE, Mackenzie HI. Observations on cyanuric acid as a source of non-protein nitrogen for sheep. *Journal of the South African Veterinary Medical Association* 1964;35(2):203–205. Mackenzie HI. Melamine for sheep. *Journal of the South African Veterinary Medical Association* 1966;37:153–157.

p. 75 *At lower doses*   Clark R. Melamine crystals in sheep. *Journal of the South African Veterinary Medical Association* 1966;37:349–351.

p. 76 *Twelve years later*   Newton GL, Utley PR. Melamine as a dietary nitrogen source for ruminants. *Journal of Animal Science* 1978;47(6):1338–1344. Broome AW. The use of non-protein nitrogen in animal feeds. In: Swan HA, Lewis D, eds. *Proceedings of the University of Nottingham School of Agriculture, Second Nutrition Conference for Feed Manufacturers.* London: J & A Churchill, 1968:92–113.

p. 76 *By the late 1970s*   See, for example, Jutzi K, Cook AM, Hütter R. The degradative pathway of the s-triazine melamine. The steps to ring cleavage. *Biochemical Journal* 1982;208(3):679–684. Shelton DR, Karns JS, McCarty GW, et al. Metabolism of melamine by *Klebsiella terragena. Applied and Environmental Microbiology* 1997;7:2832–2835.

10. Melamine: A Fraudulent Adulterant

p. 77 *Decades ago* Cattaneo P, Cantoni C. Determinazione della melammina aggiunta alle farine di origine animale. *Tecnica Molitoria,* May 1979:371–374. Cattaneo P, Cantoni C. Presenza di melammina in farina di pesce. *Tecnica Molitoria,* June 1982:17–18.

p. 79 *There's a real absence* Transcript of FDA press conference on the pet food recall, May 1, 2007, at www.fda.gov/bbs/transcripts/transcript050107.pdf. Also see Ember LR. Cause of deaths, illness in pets remains elusive. *Chemical & Engineering News,* April 4, 2007, at http://pubs.acs.org/cen/news/85/i15/8515 news7.html.

p. 79 *It is not that* Pet killer? *New Scientist,* June 9, 2007:26.

p. 79 *More surprising is that* FDA. Interim melamine and analogues safety/risk assessment, May 25, 2007, at www.cfsan.fda.gov/~dms/melamra.html.

11. How Much Melamine Was in the Pet Food?

p. 81 *If 63 mg/kg* Transcripts of FDA press conferences on contaminated animal feed, May 3 and May 30, 2007, at www.fda.gov/bbs/transcripts/transcript 050307.pdf.

p. 82 *So let's do some* Actual measurements are reported in Puschner B, Poppenga RH, Lowenstine LJ, et al. Assessment of melamine and cyanuric acid toxicity in cats. *Journal of Veterinary Diagnostic Investigation* 2007;19:616–624. The authors say the California Animal Health and Food Safety laboratory measured melamine and found up to 3,200 mg/kg in pet food. The authors do not say whether the weight refers to wet food or to dry ingredients. If wet, a 5 kg animal eating 300 grams would take in 960 mg of melamine, or 192 mg/kg of body weight. If dry, a 5 kg animal might eat 100 grams of food with 320 mg of melamine, which works out to a dose of 64 mg/kg, the amount considered safe by the FDA.

12. Mystery Solved: Cyanuric Acid

p. 84 *On April 28* Roebuck K. Humans at risk from tainted pet food? *Pittsburgh Tribune-Review,* April 20, 2007. The Michigan State scientists also identified two other melamine by-products: amilorine and amiloride. See interview with Alan Wildeman. CNN transcripts, April 30, 2007, at http://transcripts .cnn.com/transcripts/0704/30/acd.02.html. Maxie G, et al. The melamine–

cyanuric acid pet food recall. *AHL Newsletter* 2007;11(2):20. Perdigão LMA, Champness NR, Beton PH. Surface self-assembly of the cyanuric acid – melamine hydrogen bonded network. *Chemical Communications* 2006;538–540.

p. 84 *To make their studies* Kyodo News International. Pedigree brand dog food recalled in Asia after illnesses reported. *Asian Economic News,* March 15, 2004, at http://findarticles.com/p/articles/mi_moWDP/is_2004_March_15/ai _114410165. Weise E, Schmit J. Pet food scare in USA had a precursor. *USA Today,* March 10, 2008, at www.usatoday.com/news/nation/2008-03-10-pet food_N.htm. Jeong W, et al. Canine renal failure syndrome in three dogs. *Journal of Veterinary Science* 2006;7:299–301.

p. 85 *The Georgia investigators* Brown CA, Jeong K-S, Poppenga RH, et al. Outbreaks of renal failure associated with melamine and cyanuric acid in dogs and cats in 2004 and 2007. *Journal of Veterinary Diagnostic Investigation* 2007;19(5):525–531.

p. 85 *At this point, it* See Steussy L. UC Davis researchers identify toxic chemicals in pet food. *The California Aggie,* November 20, 2007.

p. 86 *To do this, she* American Veterinary Medical Association. Researchers examine contaminants in food, deaths of pets. *javmaNews,* December 1, 2007, at www.avma.org/onlnews/javma/dec07/071201c-pf.asp. Puschner B, Poppenga RH, Lowenstine LJ, et al. Assessment of melamine and cyanuric acid toxicity in cats. *Journal of Veterinary and Diagnostic Investigation* 2007;19:616–624. The pig and mice studies were not yet published at the time this book went to press.

p. 87 *As is standard practice* U.C. Davis study finds chemical combo in pet-food. *Petfood Industry.com e-newsletter,* November 20, 2007.

13. The China Connection

p. 88 *ChemNutra's very business* ChemNutra: the China source experts, at www.chemnutra.com. Weiss R, Trejos N. Crisis over pet food extracting healthy cost. *Washington Post,* May 2, 2007.

p. 89 *Reasonably making use* Xuzhou Anying Biologic Technology Development Co., Ltd. At www.fuzing.com/vci/0015040d2288/Xuzhou-Anying-Biologic-Technology-Development-CoLtd. The information about wheat gluten and ESB powder was available April 21, 2007, but has since disappeared.

p. 90 *A less benign* Barboza D. Some suspect chemical mix in pet food. *New York Times,* April 12, 2007. The Melamine Material Factory site was at www .fuzian.com, accessed on April 21, 2007.

p. 90 *At the end of March* Goldstein D. Tainted wheat gluten sold as "food grade." Huffington Post, April 1, 2007, at www.huffingtonpost.com. Chem-Nutra announces nationwide wheat gluten recall — April 3, 2007 (press release), at www.chemnutra.com/media/00001.htm. The Del Monte and Sunshine Mills announcements are at www.fda.gov/oc/opacom/hottopics/petfood .html.

p. 91 *With so much at* ChemNutra FAQ, April 15, 2007, at www.chemnutra .com/ChemNutra%20FAQ.pdf.

p. 91 *But if the business* Associated Press. Farmed fish given meal tainted with melamine. MSNBC.com, May 8, 2007, at www.msnbc.msn.com/id/ 18556690.

p. 91 *The Menu Foods version* Phillips T. Menu CEO talks recalls. *Petfood Industry,* September 2007:20–22.

p. 92 *Menu Foods, according* ChemNutra FAQ, April 15, 2007, at www .chemnutra.com/ChemNutra%20FAQ.pdf. This could have been the first time ChemNutra had direct contact with Xuzhou Anying. According to the February 2008 indictment documents cited in Chapter 20, ChemNutra had only been dealing with Suzhou Textiles.

p. 92 *On April 2* Zezima K. 22 brands of dog biscuits are added to pet food recall. *New York Times,* April 6, 2007. FDA. Import alert #99–29, detention without physical examination of all vegetable protein products from China for animal or human food use due to the presence of melamine and/or melamine analogs, July 31, 2007, at www.fda.gov/ora/fiars/ora_import_ia9929.html. Associated Press. Most wheat gluten sold inside China. *USA Today,* April 5, 2007. Manning A, MacLeod C. China denies role in pet food recall. *USA Today,* April 4, 2007. Zamiska N. Who's monitoring Chinese food exports. *Wall Street Journal,* April 9, 2007.

p. 93 *Barboza's conclusion* Barboza D, Barrionuevo A. In China, additive to animals' food is an open secret. *New York Times,* April 30, 2007. Barboza D. 2nd ingredient is suspected in pet food contamination. *New York Times,* May 9, 2007.

p. 94 *But the revelations* Barboza D. Chinese firm dodged inspection of pet food, U.S. says. *New York Times,* May 3, 2007. Zamiska N. Invoice links two Chinese firms to bad pet food. *Wall Street Journal,* May 7, 2007.

p. 95 *Suzhou Textiles, as it* The company's clothing website is www.china apparel.net/catalogs/043/058/023/default.shtml. Its pharmaceutical site is http:// wil-chem.diytrade.com. The site listed as last active on October 24, 2007, is at

www.diytrade.com/directory/global/china-manufacturers/230873/main/suzhou
_textiles_light_industry_products_arts_crafts_imp_exp_co_ltd.html.

14. More Melamine

p. 98 *Our company's management* As late as April 21, 2007, Binzhou Futian
Biology Technology Co., Ltd., Shandong, China, was at www.21food.com/
showroom/27074/productlist/s-p1.html, and Shandong Flourishing Biotechnology Co., Ltd., was referred to on the Binzhou Futian website and described
at www.fuzing.com.

p. 100 *This recall must* MacLeod C. China grapples with food-safety probe.
USA Today, April 29, 2007.

p. 100 *Later analysis* At the May 8 teleconference, the FDA said its forensic
chemists had determined that both ingredients—wheat gluten and rice protein
concentrate — were actually wheat flour adulterated with melamine and
"melamine-related compound" (presumably cyanuric acid). The intrepid *USA
Today* reporters must have learned this a day earlier. See Schmit J, Weise E.
Tainted pet food: flour, in disguise, is the culprit. *USA Today,* May 8, 2007.

p. 100 *Royal Canin, for example* Mars Petcare is at www.marspetcare.com.
Cereal Byproducts Company announces the voluntary nationwide recall of rice
protein concentrate produced in China (press release), May 4, 2007, at www
.fda.gov/oc/po/firmrecalls/cerealbyproducts05_07.html.

p. 101 *Royal Canin had to* Bause T, Prinsloo H. Namibia: pet food shock—
manufacturers recall stocks. *The Namibian* (Windhoek), April 13, 2007, at http://
allafrica.com/stores/200704130385.html. Pet-food poison from SA firm. News24,
April 19, 2007, at www.news24.com/News24/South_Africa/News/0,,2-7-1442
_2101493,00.html.

p. 101 *The travails of Blue* Schmit J. Who was watching suppliers? *USA
Today,* May 10, 2007.

p. 103 *American Nutrition* American Nutrition, Inc. responds to criticism
(press release), April 30, 2007, at www.pr.com/press-release/37367.

15. More Melamine Eaters

p. 105 *As then Assistant* Dr. Acheson must have had a busy year at the FDA.
He began 2007 as chief medical officer and director of the Office of Food
Defense, Communication and Emergency Response at the Center for Food
Safety and Applied Nutrition (CFSAN). On May 1, he was appointed assistant
commissioner for food protection. In November, he replaced Robert Brackett

as acting director of CFSAN. Early in 2008, he became associate commissioner for foods.

p. 106 *Once we knew* FDA. Transcript of FDA press conference on contaminated animal feed, May 3, 2007, at www.fda.gov/bbs/transcripts/transcript 050307.pdf.

p. 106 *On April 19* Dahlberg, CP. Chemical found in state hogs. Sacbee.com, April 20, 2007, at www.sacbee.com/101/v-print/story/158442.html. Weise E, Schmit J. Human foods to be tested for melamine. *USA Today,* April 24, 2007.

p. 108 *Because the U.S. Department* Joint news release: FDA and USDA determine swine fed adulterated product, April 26, 2007, at www.fda.gov/bbs/topics/news/2007/new01618.html.

p. 109 *Steve Miller, ChemNutra's* House Committee on Energy and Commerce, April 24, 2007, at http://energycommerce.house.gov/cmte_mtgs/110-oi-hrg .042407.food.supply.shtml. Mr. Miller's remarks are at hour 3:03. Del Monte's photographs are in documents #89–#92, November 16–18, In re: Pet Food Products Liability Litigation (MDL-1850), Justia.com Federal District Court Filings and Dockets, at http://dockets.justia.com/docket/court-njdce/case_no-1:2007 cv02867/case_id-203642.

p. 109 *On April 30* Joint update: FDA/USDA trace adulterated feed to poultry, April 30, 2007, at www.fda.gov/bbs/topics/news/2007/new01621.html.

p. 110 *In reassuring* FDA/USDA joint news release: scientists conclude very low risk to humans from food containing melamine, May 7, 2007, at www.fda .gov/bbs/topics/news/2007/new01629.html.

p. 111 *Surely chickens* Fish meant for humans fed tainted food. CNN.com, May 8, 2007, at www.cnn.com/2007/HEALTH/05/08/fish.food/index.html. Le PC. Tainted feed pulled from fish hatcheries. *Seattle Intelligencer,* May 9, 2007. Simpson S. Company recalling fish feed is testing B.C. batches. *Vancouver Sun,* May 10, 2007. FDA teleconferences May 8 and May 10 at www.fda.gov/oc/opacom/hottopics/petfood.html.

p. 111 *FDA officials again* Weiss R. FDA says quarantined hogs are safe to eat. *Washington Post,* May 16, 2007. Transcript of FDA press conference on contaminated animal feed, May 15, 2007, at www.fda.gov/bbs/transcripts/transcript 051507.pdf.

p. 112 *The FDA began* FDA. Tembec and Uniscope voluntarily recall feed ingredients, May 30, 2007, at www.fda.gov/bbs/topics/NEWS/2007/NEW01643

.html. FDA recalls melamine-tainted animal feed. CNNMoney.com, May 30, 2007. Martin A. Melamine from U.S. put in feed. *New York Times,* May 31, 2007.

p. 112 *With or without* FDA. Warning letter to Tembec, September 11, 2007, at www.fda.gov/foi/warning_letters/s6509c/htm.

16. The FDA's Response

p. 116 *A better idea* FDA. Consumer update: FDA's ongoing pet food investigation, April 16, 2007, at www.fda.gov/consumer/updates/petfoodrecallup. html. FDA Science Board. Science and mission at risk: report of the Subcommittee on Science and Technology, November 2007, at www.fda.gov/ohrms/dockets/ac/07/briefing/2007-4329b_02_01_FDA%20Report%20on%20Science%20and%20Technology.pdf.

p. 117 *Some of these problems* See transcripts of FDA teleconferences from March 19 until May 30 at www.fda.gov/oc/opacom/hottopics/petfood.html.

p. 119 *As late as November* Notes on FDA teleconference with bloggers, November 14, 2007. No transcript is available; I checked my notes by listening to a recording before the FDA removed it from the website on November 21.

p. 120 *In the meantime* FDA and AAFCO. Memorandum of understanding between the U.S. Food and Drug Administration and the Association of American Feed Control Officials, FDA record #225-07-7001, April 2007. FDA, AAFCO sign agreement on feed ingredient listing (press release), November 19, 2007, at www.fda.gov/cvm/CVM_Updates/AAFCO_MOU.htm.

p. 120 *To deal with* Zhang J. FDA weighs shift in safety checks on food imports. *Wall Street Journal,* June 14, 2007. Brackett RE. Constituent update, May 9, 2007, at www.cfsan.fda.gov/~dms/cfsupdat.html.

p. 121 *This last issue* Weise E, Schmit J. Pet food scare in USA had a precursor; Asian outbreak reported in 2004. *USA Today,* March 11, 2008, at www.usatoday.com/news/nation/2008-03-10-petfood_N.htm.

17. Repercussion #1: China's Food Safety

p. 123 *China is so large* I review the history of food safety in the United States in *Safe Food: Bacteria, Biotechnology, and Bioterrorism.* Berkeley: University of California Press, 2003.

p. 124 *What's happening halfway* Mihm S. A nation of outlaws: a century ago, that wasn't China—it was us. *Boston Globe,* August 26, 2007.

p. 124 *In the context* Madden N. Is China turning into the land of tainted products? *Advertising Age,* August 20, 2007. The quotation is attributed to Scott Silverman, regional director, Asia/Pacific, for Godfrey Q & Partners in Beijing.

p. 125 *The pet food recalls* Weiss R. Pet food chemical was from 2 firms. *Washington Post,* May 4, 2007. Clapp S. USDA warns against food counterfeiters in China. *Food Chemical News,* May 7, 2007.

p. 126 *In short order* Barboza D. China yields to inquiry on pet food. *New York Times,* April 24, 2007. MacLeod C. China grapples with food-safety probe. *USA Today,* April 29, 2007. Barboza D. Chinese executive held inquiry of tainted pet food. *New York Times,* May 4, 2007. Zamiska N. China vows crackdown on food-industry offenses. *Wall Street Journal,* May 10, 2007. Barbaza D. Food-safety crackdown in China. *New York Times,* June 28, 2007. Zamiska N. Watchdog says 20% of domestic products have quality issues. *Wall Street Journal,* July 5, 2007.

p. 126 *China's vice premier* Wu Y. China stands for quality. *Wall Street Journal,* December 11, 2007.

p. 126 *China has a huge* Barboza D. Ex-chief of China food and drug unit sentenced to death for graft. *New York Times,* May 30, 2007. Barboza D. China steps up safety efforts. *New York Times,* July 7, 2007. Barboza D. A Chinese reformer betrays his cause, and pays. *New York Times,* July 13, 2007.

p. 127 *Later that month* Barboza D, Bogdanich W. China shuts 3 companies over safety of products. *New York Times,* July 21, 2007. (The third company had shipped diethylene glycol as glycerin.) Lawrence D. China says two companies face prosecution for tainted pet food, August 27, 2007, at www.bloomberg .com.

p. 127 *Given the complicated* Lee D. China's additives on menu in U.S. *New York Times,* May 18, 2007. Scherer R, Ford P. China's grip on key food additive. *Christian Science Monitor,* July 20, 2007. As China enforced environmental and safety rules, the price of vitamin C tripled in 2007. See McNally A. Chinese vitamin C supply could be under threat, September 12, 2007, at www.food qualitynews.com/news/printNewsBis.asp?id=79691. Huang S, Gale F. China's rising fruit and vegetable exports challenge U.S. industries. USDA, February 2006, at www.ers.usda.gov/Publications/FTS/2006/02Feb/FTS32001/fts32001 .pdf. National Oceanic and Atmospheric Administration. Fishwatch—U.S. seafood facts, at www.nmfs.noaa.gov/fishwatch/trade_and_aquaculture.htm.

p. 128 *Food ingredients* Ederer P, Goldberg RA. U.S. FDA: Center for Food Safety and Applied Nutrition: Food Safety in a Globalizing World. European

Food & Agribusiness, Wageningen University, August 1, 2007. Daniszewski H. Not so made in Canada. *London Free Press,* March 15, 2008, at http://lfpress .ca/cgi-bin/publish.cgi?p=227734&s=shopping.

p. 129 *Much of our trade* USDA. Latest U.S. agricultural trade data, updated November 9, 2007, at www.ers.usda.gov/data/fatus/monthlysummary.htm. China trade statistics are at www.census.gov/foreign-trade/balance/c5700 .html.

p. 129 *The large volume* Chen W, Qiong W. China: en route to better food safety. *China View,* September 16, 2007, at http://news.xinhuanet.com/ english/2007-09/16/content_6733537.htm. Schwartz ND. Chinese goods face more tests by U.S. firms. *New York Times,* July 1, 2007.

p. 130 *The safety of pet foods* See Morrison WM. China-U.S. trade issues: CRS report for Congress, updated October 3, 2007, at www.fas.org/sgp/crs/ row/RL33536.pdf. Weisman SR. Food safety joins issues at U.S.-China talks. *New York Times,* May 23, 2007. Miller JW, Batson A. EU toughens stance in dealings with China. *Wall Street Journal,* November 29, 2007.

p. 130 *In late May* USDA and HHS. Fact sheet: Actions requested of the People's Republic of China by the U.S. government to address the safety of food and feed, May 24, 2007, at www.usda.gov/wps/portal/!ut/p/_s.7_0_A/7 _0_1OB?contentidonly=true&contentid=2007/05/0152.xml. China says some U.S. goods didn't meet safety standards. *New York Times,* June 9, 2007. Zamiska N, Spencer J. China faces a new worry: heavy metals in the food. *Wall Street Journal,* July 2, 2007.

p. 131 *In the midst* Martin A. F.D.A. curbs sale of five seafoods farmed in China. *New York Times,* June 29, 2007. Barboza D. China vows food-safety changes. *New York Times,* June 30, 2007. Barboza D. A slippery, writhing dispute. *New York Times,* July 3, 2007. China blames media for food health scares. Reuters, July 16, 2007, at www.msnbc.msn.com/id/19787723. Today's debate: product safety. *USA Today,* July 10, 2007. Dyer G. Beijing concedes flaws in food safety system. *Financial Times,* July 10, 2007.

p. 131 *In response to* Batson A. China tightens local oversight. *Wall Street Journal,* August 10, 2007. Lipton E. China plans to inspect more food. *New York Times,* August 16, 2007. Barboza D. China acts to cleanse reputation. *New York Times,* September 5, 2007. Zamiska N. Beijing challenges U.S. over product safety. *Wall Street Journal,* September 11, 2007. MacLeod C. China details new food-quality measures. *USA Today,* September 13, 2007. Barboza D. 774 arrests in China over safety. *New York Times,* October 30, 2007.

p. 132 *In November* Zhe Z. Draft food safety law approved. *ChinaDaily,* November 1, 2007, at www.chinadaily.com.cn/china/2007-11/01/content_6221398 .htm. Barboza D. China moves to improve quality of its seafood. *New York Times,* December 28, 2007. Blanchard B. China says food safety push a complete success. *Guardian Unlimited,* January 14, 2008, at http://uk.reuters.com/article/worldnews/idukpek35091620080114. Bogdanich W. Blood thinner might be tied to more deaths. *New York Times,* February 29, 2008, at www.nytimes.com/2008/02/29/us/29heparin.html?scp=2&sq=chinese+heparin&st=nyt.

18. Repercussion #2: The China Backlash

p. 133 *Back in the United* Hubbard and Dingell are quoted in Ederer P, Goldberg RA. U.S. FDA: Center for Food Safety and Applied Nutrition: Food Safety in a Globalizing World. European Food & Agribusiness, Wageningen University, August 1, 2007:4. Paulson's quote is in Weisman SR. U.S. to pressure China on food and product safety at coming trade talks. *New York Times,* December 7, 2007. See Tourtellotte B. Health food maker promotes "China-free" products. Reuters, July 6, 2007. Barboza D. An export boom suddenly facing a quality crisis. *New York Times,* May 18, 2007. Barboza D. When fakery turns fatal. *New York Times,* June 5, 2007.

p. 133 *Nevertheless, labels* Roberts S. To Beijing games, bring your own. *New York Times,* July 10, 2007. Shpigel B. Wary of food, U.S. Olympians plan a big delivery to China. *New York Times,* February 9, 2008. Schmit J. Trader Joe's to exclude some food imports from China. *USA Today,* February 11, 2008. Hirsch J. Grocer curtails China imports. *Los Angeles Times,* February 12, 2008.

p. 134 *Fears of the hazards* See the website of Sustain: The Alliance for Better Food and Farming at www.sustainweb.org, and Halweil B, *Eat Here: Home-grown Pleasures in a Global Supermarket.* New York: W. W. Norton, 2004.

p. 135 *The origin of many* The origins of COOL in the United States are described in General Accounting Office, *Country-of-Origin Labeling: Opportunities for USDA and Industry to Implement Challenging Aspects of the New Law* (GAO-03-780), August 2003, at www.gao.gov. For basic information, see USDA at www.ams.usda.gov/cool. Also see News from the House Agriculture Committee. House Agriculture Committee passes groundbreaking farm bill, July 20, 2007, at http://agriculture.house.gov/list/press/agriculture_dem/pr_072007_FarmBill_Passage.html.

p. 136 *From 2002 to 2007* Nestle M. *What to Eat.* New York: Farrar, Straus & Giroux, 2006. The Grocery Manufacturers of America merged in 2007 with the Food Products Association (formerly the National Food Processors Association) to form the Grocery Manufacturers Association. See www.gmaonline .org.

p. 137 *Congress may have been* Clapp S. Zogby poll shows overwhelming support for COOL, and Senators voice support for including COOL in farm·bill, *Food Chemical News,* August 20 and October 15, 2007.

p. 138 *to a cost-effective* Interagency Working Group on Import Safety. Protecting the American consumer every step of the way: a strategic framework for import safety, September 10, 2007, at www.importsafety.gov/report/report .pdf.

p. 138 *I have no idea* Murphy J. GMA embraces tougher mandatory standards for food importers. *Food Chemical News,* September 24, 2007. Grocery Manufacturers Association unveils action plan for strengthening imported food safety (undated press release), at www.gmaonline.org/news/docs/News Release.cfm?DocID=1772. Merle R. Food firms want FDA to oversee imports. *Washington Post,* September 19, 2007. Interagency Working Group on Import Safety. Action plan for import safety: report to the president, November 6, 2007, at www.importsafety.gov/report/actionplan.pdf.

p. 140 *On the international* Wu Y. China stands for quality. *Wall Street Journal,* December 11, 2007.

p. 140 *The dialogue* Weisman S. China agrees to post U.S. safety officials in its food factories. *New York Times,* December 12, 2007. Leow J, Zhang J. China, U.S. pacts close product-safety loophole. *Wall Street Journal,* December 12, 2007, at http://online.wsj.com/article/SB119736127724320701.html. The quote is from former FDA associate commissioner William Hubbard.

p. 141 *The General Accounting* See, for example, Durbin: GAO report confirms need for a single food safety agency, February 22, 2005, at http://durbin .senate.gov/record.cfm?id=233497. DeWaal CS, Plunkett DW. Building a modern food safety system: for FDA regulated foods, Center for Science in the Public Interest, November 2007, at www.cspinet.org/new/pdf/fswhitepaper. pdf. Heller L. Lawmakers renew call for single food safety agency, February 19, 2007, at www.foodnavigator-usa.com/news/ng.asp?n=74322-food-safety -safe-food-act. Clinton proposes new safety measures to ensure imported products are safe for American families (press release), November 20, 2007, at www .iowapolitics.com/index.iml?Article=111122. Salvage B. John Edwards lists positions on food safety, imports. MeatPoultry.com, December 11, 2007. Each beef recall leads to more calls for a single food agency. See The biggest beef recall ever (editorial). *New York Times,* February 21, 2008.

19. Repercussion #3: The FDA in Crisis

p. 143 *If the FDA* Ederer P, Goldberg RA. U.S. FDA: Center for Food Safety and Applied Nutrition: Food Safety in a Globalizing World. European Food & Agribusiness, Wageningen University, August 1, 2007. Mr. Hubbard retired from his position as FDA commissioner for policy and planning in 2005.

p. 144 *The regulatory framework* Ederer and Goldberg, U.S. FDA.

p. 144 *That paradigm* FDA. Spinach and E. coli outbreak (home page), at www.fda.gov/oc/opacom/hottopics/spinach.html.

p. 145 *First the history* On the irrationality, history, and politics of the U.S. food safety system, see Nestle M. *Safe Food: Bacteria, Biotechnology, and Bioterrorism.* Berkeley: University of California Press, 2003.

p. 146 *More resources* USDA. What share of U.S. consumed food is imported? *Amber Waves,* February 2008. Harris G. For F.D.A., a major backlog overseas. *New York Times,* January 29, 2008. Government Accountability Office. Federal oversight of food safety: FDA's food protection plan proposes positive first steps, but capacity to carry them out is critical (GAO-08-435T), January 29, 2008.

p. 147 *After September 11* Pulaski A. Pet crisis spotlights gaps in food safety. *The Oregonian,* April 28, 2007. Schmit J. U.S. food imports outrun FDA resources. *USA Today,* March 19, 2007. Barrionuevo A. Food imports often escape scrutiny. *New York Times,* May 1, 2007. Martin A, Palmer G. China not sole source of dubious food. *New York Times,* July 12, 2007.

p. 147 *The low inspection* FDA Science Board. Science and mission at risk: report of the Subcommittee on Science and Technology, November 2007, at www.fda.gov/ohrms/dockets/ac/07/briefing/2007-4329b_02_01_FDA%20 Report%20on%20Science%20and%20Technology.pdf. The report was adopted by the Science Board on December 3.

p. 149 *In reviewing* Union of Concerned Scientists. FDA scientists pressured to exclude, alter findings, July 20, 2006, at www.ucsusa.org/news/press_release/ fda-scientists-pressured.html. Zegart D. The gutting of the civil service. *The Nation,* November 20, 2006, at www.thenation.com/doc/20061120/zegart/2.

p. 150 *The highly political* FDA. Food protection plan: an integrated strategy for protecting the nation's food supply, November 2007, at www.fda.gov/oc/ initiatives/advance/food/plan.pdf. The plan was announced at a press conference on November 6. See HHS unveils plan to strengthen, update food safety efforts, at www.hhs.gov/news/press/2007pres/11/pr20071106a.html.

p. 152 *I was by no* Clapp S. FDA and GMA officials quizzed on import safety plans. *Food Chemical News,* November 19, 2007:1,9. Zhang J. Plan for food safety criticized at hearing. *Wall Street Journal,* December 5, 2007.

p. 153 *The pet food scandal* Ederer and Goldberg, U.S. FDA.

p. 153 *As I mentioned* I review the science and politics of mad cow disease in the final chapter of *Safe Food* and in the chapter on meat safety in *What to Eat* (New York: Farrar, Straus & Giroux, 2006). Also see Rampton S, Stauber J. *Mad Cow U.S.A.* Monroe, ME: Common Courage Press, 2004; and Schwartz M. *How the Cows Turned Mad.* Berkeley: University of California Press, 2004. See Cornell University College of Veterinary Medicine. Veterinary information brief: mad cow disease and cats, November 15, 2006, at www.vet.cornell .edu/fhc/news/madcow.htm. Statistics on spongiform encephalopathies in cats are from the British Department for Environment, Food and Rural Affairs at www.defra.gov.uk/animalh/bse/statistics/incidence.html. No cases have been reported in cats since 2001.

p. 154 *consumers and the* FDA Science Board. Science and mission at risk: report of the Subcommittee on Science and Technology, November 2007, at www.fda.gov/ohrms/dockets/ac/07/briefing/2007-4329b_02_01_FDA%20 Report%20on%20Science%20and%20Technology.pdf.

p. 154 *This brings us* You're eating that? (editorial). *New York Times,* November 26, 2007. Also, Ederer and Goldberg, U.S. FDA.

p. 154 *By December 2007* Morgan & Myers. Many consumers trust activists and grocers for food information (news release), December 5, 2007, at www .morganmyers.com/home_p.htm.

20. Repercussion #4: Pet Food Politics

p. 156 *Advocates for* Standard safety procedures are collectively called HACCP—Hazard Analysis and Critical Control Point with Pathogen Reduction. They require food companies to identify places in production systems where hazards might occur (analysis), take steps to prevent hazards at those places (critical control points), and monitor to make sure the steps were taken and worked (pathogen reduction). See the FDA's HACCP website at www .cfsan.fda.gov/~lrd/haccp.html.

p. 156 *We do feel that* Ekedahl D. Testimony before the Senate Committee on Appropriations, Subcommittee on Agriculture, Rural Development, Food and Drug Administration, and Related Agencies, April 12, 2007, at http:// appropriations.senate.gov/hearings.cfm.

p. 157 *In September, Congress* Food and Drug Administration Amendments Act of 2007, Public Law 110-85, 110th Congress (September 27, 2007), at www .govtrack.us/congress/bill.xpd?bill=h110-3580.

p. 157 *The government of* The Canadian Food Inspection Agency's activities and actions can be accessed at www.inspection.gc.ca/english/toce.shtml. See Melamine in imported products at www.inspection.gc.ca/english/fssa/concen/ specif/vegproe.shtml. A year after Menu Foods scandal, pet food off the radar of regulators. *The Canadian Press,* March 15, 2008, at http://canadianpress .google.com/article/ALeqM5jpnJ3tN-OsNj2L24mfrSeIjoaJkA.

p. 158 *In the immediate* Pet Food Institute. Advertisement, *USA Today,* April 12, 2007. For an outline of the public relations strategy, see Bush M. Pet food industry unites in crisis. *PR Week,* May 17, 2007.

p. 160 *Create some kind* Waddell L. A galaxy of PR woe. *Newsweek,* December 14, 2007, at www.newsweek.com/id/78044/output/print.

p. 160 *If the impetus* Lummis D. Selling safety. *Petfood Industry,* September 2007:24−27.

p. 161 *On average, sales* The March 16 and March 30 Hill's recall notices are on the FDA's melamine recall website at www.fda.gov/oc/opacom/hottopics/ petfood.html. Henderson D. Pet food makers working to bring trust back to the table. *Boston Globe,* May 22, 2007. Neff J. In the wake of pet-food crisis, Iams sales plummet nearly 17%. *Advertising Age,* May 14, 2007. Schmit J. Pet-food industry feels side effects of recall. *USA Today,* August 11, 2007.

p. 161 *By the end of* See Update 1-Menu Foods swings to loss on pet food recall woes. Reuters, February 13, 2008, at www.reuters.com/articlePrint?article ID=USN1337018020080213. Menu Foods posts $62M net loss for 2007. *Farm Business Communications,* February 14, 2008, at www.albertafarmexpress .ca/issues/ISArticle.asp?id=80172&issue=02142008&story_id=&PC=FBC. PetSmart still recovering from pet food recall—CEO. Reuters, September 6, 2007, at www.reuters.com/articlePrint?articleID=USN0630201220070906.

p. 161 *Within days of* Pet Valu a possible target in tainted-pet-food suit. Thestar.com, September 19, 2007, at www.thestar.com/printArticle/258283. Malanga S. Pet plaintiffs. *Wall Street Journal,* May 9, 2007.

p. 162 *Some legal authorities* Walker AF. Ontario courts award compensation for emotional distress associated with the loss of a pet. *The Canadian Veterinary Journal* 2007;48(9):967−969, at www.pubmedcentral.nih.gov/articlerender.fcgi ?artid=1950104.

p. 162 *Lawyers also*   Maltzman Foreman. Class action lawsuit against pet food companies and retailers, May 15, 2007, at www.mflegal.com/petfoodlawsuit. Menu Foods Income Fund. Multi-district mediation produces agreeement in principle, April 1, 2008, at www.marketwire.com/mw/release.do?id=838913. Details of the case are at In re: Pet Food Products Liability Litigation (MDL-1850), Justia.com Federal District Court Filings and Dockets, at http://dockets.justia.com/docket/court-njdce/case_no-1:2007cv02867/case_id-203642.

p. 163 *As it happened*   E-mail, November 5, 2007.

p. 164 *Indeed, some instructive*   FDA investigation leads to several indictments for importing contaminated ingredients used in pet food (press release), February 6, 2008, at www.fda.gov/bbs/topics/news/2008/new01792.html. See Schmit J, Weise E. Three firms indicted in pet-food recall case. *USA Today,* February 6, 2008, at www.usatoday.com/money/industries/manufacturing/2008-02-06-pet-food-deaths_n.htm?loc=interstitialskip. This last article provides links to the federal prosecutor's statement and to the indictment documents pertaining to the Millers and ChemNutra and to Xuzhou Anying and Suzhou Textiles.

p. 165 *Before Blue Buffalo*   Goldman A. Sniffing out answers in pet food scandal. *Los Angeles Times,* July 1, 2007. Flaim D. Raw facts on another feeding option. *Newsday,* March 20, 2007. Turner D. Pet owners are making dog and cat food. Yahoo! News, April 3, 2007. Neff J. Pet-food crisis a boon to organic players. *Advertising Age,* April 8, 2007. Zezima K. On the trail of wholesome pet dinners. *New York Times,* April 11, 2007. Mintel Oxygen. Pet food and supplies — US — August 2007: supply structure, at http://oxygen.mintel.com (by subscription or through business libraries).

p. 166 *Nevertheless, the recalls*   See Pet Food Products Safety Alliance at www.pfpsa.org/faq.html. Top dog: organic and natural pet food sales soar in wake of China scandal. *Nutrition Business Journal,* July/August 2007:26–27.

p. 166 *The companies that*   Phillips T. Natural Balance rebounds: 3 keys. *Petfood Industry,* February 2008:26–29. See www.naturalbalanceinc.com. Castor & Pollux is at www.castorpolluxpet.com.

p. 168 *Pet Food Express*   Pet Food Express is at petfoodexpress.com. What it will not sell is at www.petfoodexpress.com/petfood/default.asp?pageid=80 &Section=About. See McPhee D. Pet Food Express takes top honors. Pet Product News International (undated), at www.petproductnews.com/top_stories/ROTY-Pet-Food-Express-0709.aspx.

p. 168 *Such sentiments are* Kerns N. Full disclosure: we've upped the ante for this year's dry dog food review. *The Whole Dog Journal* 2008;11(2):3–11.

p. 169 *The American College* American College of Veterinary Nutrition. ACVN statement on pet food recalls, April 6, 2007, at www.acvn.org/site/view/92016_ACVNPetFoodRecalls.pml.

p. 171 *The pet recall sites* Weise E. Pet-food scandal ignites blogosphere, and pet-owning bloggers mobilize on food front. *USA Today,* June 5, 2007. The victims' site is http://menufoodsvictims.blogspot.com. Keith C. Pet food recall panel—and your vote counts! Pet Connection, August 22, 2007, at www.pet connection.com/blog/2007/08/22/1879.

p. 172 *Fifteen cats* Keith C. Bigger than you think: the story behind the pet food recall. *San Francisco Chronicle,* April 3, 2007. Keith C. The pet food recall: one year later, has anything changed? *San Francisco Chronicle,* March 15, 2008.

Appendix: The Melamine Recalls List

p. 175 *The FDA's final list* FDA. Search for pet food recalls. Updated October 31, 2007, at www.accessdata.fda.gov/scripts/petfoodrecall/#All. The FDA's melamine recall page (updated February 6, 2008) is at www.fda.gov/oc/opacom/hottopics/petfood.html.

p. 176 *The FDA site and that* American Veterinary Medical Association. Pet food recalls (home page), updated June 13, 2007, but provides information about recalls through August 22, 2007, at www.avma.org/aa/petfoodrecall/default.asp.

LIST OF TABLES
AND FIGURES

Tables

Figures

ACKNOWLEDGMENTS

As with all such projects, many people deserve praise and thanks. For investigative journalism at its best, I am especially indebted to Elizabeth Weise and Julie Schmit of *USA Today,* David Barboza of *The New York Times,* Christie Keith and Gina Spadafori of Pet Connection, Carrie Peyton Dahlberg of the *Sacramento Bee,* and Karen Roebuck of the *Pittsburgh Tribune-Review.* Much of this account is based on their work. I also owe thanks to the anonymous staff at the FDA who produced and maintain the agency's melamine and pet food websites; these provide an invaluable archive of documents related to the recalls as well as a great public service.

I thank Jim Harkness of the Institute for Agriculture and Trade Policy for allowing me to plagiarize his Chihuahua idea for the title; Celia Sack and Paula Harris of Noe Valley Pet Company for the gift of a recalled cat food; my Canadian cousin, Ted Zittell, for his explanation of the history of Menu Foods; and my neighbors Lynn Russell and Irv Schenkler, for the loan of their Samoyed, Klara, and for the introduction to Klara's expert trainer and photographer, Lori Sash-Gail. I am grateful to Neal Barnard, Rose Levy Beranbaum, Robert Brackett, Dave Carter, George Daston, Ellen Fried, Alan Goldberg, Francis Kallfelz, Nancy Kerns, Michael Levy, Terry Lim, Ralph Loglisci, Don Smith, Fred Tripp, Kenneth Wexler, and Lisa Young for contributing ideas, information, referrals, or documents, and to Claudia Kawczynska of *The Bark* for welcoming Mal Nesheim and me into her magazine's editorial realm.

For research assistance on this project, I gratefully acknowledge the superb work of Brelyn Johnson at NYU and Heather Catherine Inglis at Cornell; Heather's impressively referenced timeline of the recall was the basis of much of this book. For keeping my electronic life in order, I am forever indebted to Sheldon Oliver Watts. For cheerfully providing assistance in countless ways, I thank Andy Bellatti, Lisa Kroin, and Kelli Ranieri. Much appreciation to Andy Bellatti, Maya Joseph, and Rebecca Nestle for sharp-eyed review of the galleys.

For their ongoing support of this project, special thanks to my agent, Lydia Wills, and to Rebecca Saletan, the editor of Mal Nesheim's and my forthcoming book with Harcourt, *What Pets Eat.*

It has been an absolute pleasure to work with the skilled team at University of California Press—project manager Dore Brown, copy editor Jan Spauschus, and cover designer Lia Tjandra. I especially thank my dear editor, Stan Holwitz—this is our third book together. To my colleagues in the Department of Nutrition, Food Studies, and Public Health at NYU and to Dean Mary Brabeck, I offer infinite appreciation for making my work possible under the most pleasant of circumstances. Last but most definitely not least, I thank Malden Nesheim for his wise counsel, scientific acumen, knowledge of animal nutrition, generosity in reading and commenting on multiple iterations of this manuscript, and delightful company.

INDEX

Page letters with the letter *t* indicate pages with tables and page numbers with the letter *f* indicate pages with figures.

Text:	11/15 Granjon
Display:	Gotham, Helvetica Rounded
Compositor:	BookMatters, Berkeley
Indexer:	Marcia Carlson
Illustrator:	Bill Nelson
Printer/Binder:	Maple-Vail Book Manufacturing Group